Overcoming Common Problems Series

Overcoming Common Problems Series

Living with Type 1 Diabetes
Dr Tom Smith

Losing a Parent
Fiona Marshall

Making Sense of Trauma: How to tell your story
Dr Nigel C. Hunt and Dr Sue McHale

Menopause: The drug-free way
Dr Julia Bressan

Menopause in Perspective
Philippa Pigache

Motor Neurone Disease: A family affair
Dr David Oliver

The Multiple Sclerosis Diet Book
Tessa Buckley

Overcome Your Fear of Flying
Professor Robert Bor, Dr Carina Eriksen and
Margaret Oakes

Overcoming Anger: When anger helps and when it hurts
Dr Windy Dryden

Overcoming Anorexia
Professor J. Hubert Lacey, Christine Craggs-Hinton
and Kate Robinson

Overcoming Anxiety
Dr Windy Dryden

Overcoming Back Pain
Dr Tom Smith

Overcoming Emotional Abuse
Susan Elliot-Wright

Overcoming Fear with Mindfulness
Deborah Ward

Overcoming Gambling: A guide for problem and compulsive gamblers
Philip Mawer

Overcoming Jealousy
Dr Windy Dryden

Overcoming Loneliness
Alice Muir

Overcoming Low Self-esteem with Mindfulness
Deborah Ward

Overcoming Stress
Professor Robert Bor, Dr Carina Eriksen and Dr
Sara Chaudry

Overcoming Worry and Anxiety
Dr Jerry Kennard

The Pain Management Handbook: Your personal guide
Neville Shone

The Panic Workbook
Dr Carina Eriksen, Professor Robert Bor and
Margaret Oakes

Physical Intelligence: How to take charge of your weight
Dr Tom Smith

Post-Traumatic Stress Disorder: Recovery after accident and disaster
Professor Kevin Gournay

Reducing Your Risk of Dementia
Dr Tom Smith

The Self-esteem Journal
Alison Waines

Stammering: Advice for all ages
Renée Byrne and Louise Wright

Stress-related Illness
Dr Tim Cantopher

The Stroke Survival Guide
Mark Greener

Ten Steps to Positive Living
Dr Windy Dryden

Therapy for Beginners: How to get the best out of counselling
Professor Robert Bor, Sheila Gill and Anne Stokes

Think Your Way to Happiness
Dr Windy Dryden and Jack Gordon

Transforming Eight Deadly Emotions into Healthy Ones
Dr Windy Dryden

The Traveller's Good Health Guide: A guide for those living, working and travelling internationally
Dr Ted Lankester

Treat Your Own Knees
Jim Johnson

Treating Arthritis: More ways to a drug-free life
Margaret Hills

Treating Arthritis: The drug-free way
Margaret Hills and Christine Horner

Treating Arthritis: The supplements guide
Julia Davies

Treating Arthritis Diet Book
Margaret Hills

Treating Arthritis Exercise Book
Margaret Hills and Janet Horwood

Understanding High Blood Pressure
Dr Shahid Aziz and Dr Zara Aziz

Understanding Obsessions and Compulsions
Dr Frank Tallis

Understanding Yourself and Others: Practical ideas from the world of coaching
Bob Thomson

When Someone You Love Has Dementia
Susan Elliot-Wright

When Someone You Love Has Depression: A handbook for family and friends
Barbara Baker

The Whole Person Recovery Handbook
Emma Drew

Overcoming Common Problems

Beating Insomnia
Without really trying

DR TIM CANTOPHER

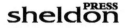
sheldon **PRESS**

First published in Great Britain in 2016

Sheldon Press
36 Causton Street
London SW1P 4ST
www.sheldonpress.co.uk

British Library Cataloguing-in-Publication Data
A catalogue record for this book is available from the British Library

ISBN 978–1–84709–258–8
eBook ISBN 978–1–84709–259–5

Typeset by Fakenham Prepress Solutions, Fakenham, Norfolk NR21 8NN
First printed in Great Britain by Ashford Colour Press
Subsequently digitally reprinted in Great Britain

eBook by Fakenham Prepress Solutions, Fakenham, Norfolk NR21 8NN

Produced on paper from sustainable forests

To Laura, whose sleep I disrupt

Contents

Acknowledgements

I am indebted to my excellent colleagues, Drs Paul Bailey, Mike Bristow, Laurence Church, Ian Drever, Eileen Feeney, John Hook, Saad Khalaf and Mark Slaney, for their time and advice, which enabled me to hide my areas of ignorance.

Note to the reader

The advice in this book is intended as a general guide, and not as a substitute for the medical advice of your doctor. Always consult your own doctor for advice on individual medical issues and requirements, particularly with respect to any symptoms that may require diagnosis or medical attention.

Introduction

Jane is worried.

> I've got a really important presentation tomorrow. My boss and most of
> the board will be there and they will all be judging my performance. I'd
> better be on top form. My future career is on the line. In fact, if it goes
> badly I'll probably be fired. I'll never get another job as they'll give me
> a lousy reference and word will get around that I'm no good. Nobody
> dates a loser. I'll probably end up dying alone and destitute in a ditch.
> Unless I can be a star tomorrow. I'll have to get a really good night's
> sleep. Everything depends on it.

Or so she thinks. She's wrong on many counts, but she's already set
up the beginnings of a self-fulfilling, if hyperbolic, prophecy.

Jane goes to bed two hours earlier than normal at 9 p.m., half an
hour after finishing supper. She has skipped her usual early evening
jog round the block, to save time. She's already had a vat of strong
coffee through the day at work to be razor sharp while working on
what she's going to say tomorrow. She does some last-minute prep
on her presentation in bed and then turns the light out. She's really
wired, with a host of worries and ideas all jostling for space in her
brain.

Top of the list is: 'I must get to sleep.' What? Are you kidding
me? You've got no chance. Jane, even if you hadn't got it all wrong
from the moment you got to work, this injunction alone is enough
to ensure a horrible night of insomnia. Sleep is a process dictated
by circadian rhythms and arousal level (I'll explain what I mean
by this later), not by determination. You can't *make* yourself sleep.

Now it's 10 p.m. and Jane is even more worried. She usually goes
to sleep within 15 minutes. Something is wrong. As the next hour
passes she experiences a sense of gathering dread. She tries not to
think about anything, but the thoughts just keep popping into her
head, whether she likes it or not. By 11 p.m. she's beside herself.
This is her normal bedtime and all the benefit of an early night has
been lost. Midnight, and sleep is as far away as the moon, but Jane
stays in bed. She can't get up because she's got to sleep. But all that

happens is that the silence and darkness of the bedroom is filled with her despair. She's doomed, she'll never be able to do it; it'll be a disaster. As dawn breaks, it finds her a sweaty heap of misery.

Jane finally drops off at 5.30 a.m. At 6.15 a.m. the alarm goes off and she almost sleeps through it. She's exhausted.

By the time she gets to work she's befuddled. She's last on the agenda of the board meeting, and an hour into it, while the Head of Compliance is presenting his new policy on form-filling, she starts snoring. She's woken up by her boss to do her presentation and promptly has a panic attack. It goes from bad to worse and in the end the CEO cuts her off early to move on to 'any other business'.

That was bad: humiliating and definitely a short-term blip in Jane's rise through the company, there's no denying that. However, I would just point out that Jane doesn't lose her job, she doesn't go bankrupt and she doesn't suffer a life of desolate solitude.

Jane is an amalgam of many of the mistakes made by my patients over the years, and we can learn a lot from her. She has experienced (and caused) the commonest type of insomnia (stress-induced), which happens to the good honest triers of the world. While not sleeping was far from ideal, in fact it wasn't this which was the main factor in undermining her performance; it was her fear of not sleeping. Worry is very debilitating, much more than one night's poor sleep. If Jane had kept to her usual routine, accepted that she may have an interrupted night because of nervous anticipation, shrugged her shoulders and experienced whatever transpired without trying to wrestle it to the ground, she would have been fine. In truth, these folks usually end up achieving their aims in the long term. Success isn't the problem but it is achieved at the cost of sleep issues and a host of other stress-related symptoms.

This isn't to say that insomnia isn't a problem; it is. One night of insomnia is miserable, lonely and wearing. Chronic insomnia is a very debilitating symptom with potential consequences for health. But there are things which you can do to help matters and, if stress is at the root of your sleep problems, avoiding Jane's mistakes may make a huge difference.

There are lots of other causes of insomnia which I will cover in this book, together with a few other problems which stop sleep from doing what we want it to – that is, to refresh and regenerate us. But if there is one take-away message I would like you to gain from these pages, it is summed up by a slight tweak to the words of the song by Frankie Goes to Hollywood: 'Relax . . . if you want to *sleep*.'

1

Does insomnia matter?

Yes, it certainly does. It's easy for those who sleep well to dismiss insomnia as a trivial gripe, but the truth is that it is one of the major afflictions of the modern world, being responsible for a great deal of lost productivity, accidents and suffering. About one in three of us report sleep problems and around one in ten complain of daytime symptoms as a result. There's a lot of it about and it tends to become more of a problem as you get older.

The relationship between insomnia and disease is difficult to tease out, because illness leads to insomnia, but maybe the reverse is also true. Insomnia has been linked to anxiety, major depression, cognitive disturbance, high blood pressure, heart disease, diabetes and increased proneness to infections. However, stress, which predisposes to these conditions, also is a cause of insomnia, so the cause–effect link isn't totally clear. Disease causes stress, which causes insomnia.

What is clear is that insomnia can cause great suffering. Being awake when others are asleep, as any insomniac will tell you, causes great stress, which in turn increases proneness to disease. What is also clear, though, is that one or a few nights of insomnia or poor sleep isn't going to kill you or do you permanent harm, so long as you don't drive or operate heavy machinery when sleep-deprived. This is a problem which you have time to resolve; whether you sleep well tonight or not isn't as crucial as it feels. Whether you sleep adequately over the next few years is.

Sleeplessness is important and is worth fixing. Your sleep can be improved. This is going to need you to make some changes in your life, to learn techniques and to practise them regularly. You are going to need to be persistent and patient. Results may take some time to appear.

Above all, you are going to have to *stop trying to sleep*. Sleep improves over time through doing the right things, not by you gritting your teeth and wrestling your wakefulness to the ground. This is counter-intuitive to many of us. We were taught as children that if you try hard, you will succeed. It's the effort which counts. This doesn't work for sleep. It's more like training a kitten – you can't force it to do what you want; you just have to keep doing the same things consistently and you get there in the end.

Taking a phlegmatic view of insomnia is also difficult for exactly the reason I gave at the beginning of this chapter. It is important and we don't tend to shrug our shoulders at things which have such major potential consequences. But we do need to achieve this calm acceptance of insomnia in the short term if we are to prevail in the long term. Top sports stars all know this principle. They all practise really hard and concentrate well, but then in the game they don't strain too much or worry about the result, as they know that just makes them tense and impairs performance. The apparently effortless excellence of the champion comes from doing the right things over and over again in practice. That is how your insomnia will be overcome too.

So maybe chronic insomnia can cause health problems, but so what? There isn't any point in worrying about what you can't control. As I have explained, you can't immediately control insomnia. But stress, now there's a real worry. If it doesn't sound too ridiculous, you should worry about the fact that you worry so much. The evidence that long-term anxiety causes a whole host of health problems is incontrovertible, as is the fact that it makes existing problems, such as pain, much worse. The causal link between anxiety and heart disease, strokes, bowel diseases, inflammatory conditions and some cancers is well established. Reducing our anxiety would improve our long-term health as clearly as exercise and good diet. It would also allow us to perform better in whatever we are doing. You are worrying about your insomnia impairing your work performance, risking your physical health and making yourself feel bad, when in truth your stressful lifestyle and tendency to worry have a far greater influence on these factors.

We can do something fairly quickly about stress and anxiety. This, in my opinion, is where you should start to deal with your insomnia. I will come to the details of how to manage anxiety later on, but I would suggest you go to Chapter 9 for the relaxation exercise (page 48) and the section on mindfulness (page 51) and start practising these strategies straight away. There is also no reason to delay looking critically at your lifestyle. The chances are that you are going to have to make some tough decisions and changes if you are going to start leading your life at a healthy level of arousal compatible with good sleep. Start thinking about these issues now. Why wait?

Incidentally, you will see the word 'arousal' crop up quite often in this book. I'm not referring to sexual arousal, but to how hot you are running. You could use the words 'stress', 'tension', 'alertness', 'excitement' or 'enjoyment', as they all refer to how switched on your nervous system is, depending on whether the experience is pleasant or unpleasant. Your body doesn't know the difference and is unlikely to allow sleep whatever the reason for your high level of arousal.

So I want to emphasize this point: sleep is important, but not necessarily tonight. It is the 'given', held by so many of my patients, that 'I must sleep well (now)' which is the single most destructive factor against their sleeping. Here is the bad news: you probably won't sleep well, not yet. There is no quick fix, other than medication (of which more in a later chapter) for insomnia. You need to come to terms with that as a starting point. If you have short-term insomnia, it is miserable for you but it isn't disastrous. If you have long-term insomnia, it is a serious problem and quite disabling, but here is the good news: if you are realistic, patient and follow any advice given by your doctor and the advice in this book, there is a very good chance that your sleep will improve greatly over time.

Your doctor has an important role here. There are many different causes of insomnia (see Chapter 4), some easily treatable. If there are medical or other causes of your poor sleep, they need to be found and dealt with.

2

How sleep works

Stages of sleep

I introduced the concept of arousal in the previous chapter. Your level of arousal varies throughout the day and night. At the highest level of arousal, you are highly alert and, if you are a calm person, at your peak. If your peak levels are higher, you may be excited or stressed; even, if you are an anxious person, panicky. At the lowest level of arousal in your 24-hour cycle, you are deeply asleep.

The point here is that your graph of arousal through 24 hours will look very like mine, even if I'm as cool as a cucumber and a good sleeper while you may be an insomniac prone to worrying. Your graph is just shifted upwards throughout the day and night compared with mine (see Figure 2.1).

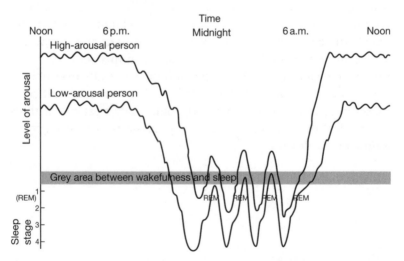

Figure 2.1 Arousal level over 24 hours in low- and high-arousal subjects

4

There is no clear division between wakefulness and sleep. Drowsiness shades into light sleep without a break. Through the night, the deepness of sleep varies, typically following a repeating pattern of around 90 minutes in length. There are five levels of sleep. At the beginning of the night, a person passes from drowsing, through level 1, to levels 2, 3 and so on, then the process is reversed with the level of sleep becoming lighter, even possibly emerging into wakefulness briefly, before the cycle begins again.

Stage 1 sleep typically lasts five to ten minutes. Muscles become relaxed and twitching or jerks sometimes occur. While the person is asleep, she may be vaguely aware of her surroundings, noises, voices and such like. It is this awareness which often persuades the light sleeper that she has been awake throughout the night, when objective observation reveals that she has been asleep much of the time. I call the grey area from drowsiness through stage 1 sleep 'drowsing'.

Stage 2 typically lasts around 20 minutes in adults who sleep well. Movement slows to a stop, body temperature falls and the heart slows. Other metabolic functions also slow down and stay slowed for much of the night, though metabolic rate rises and falls to an extent with the depth of sleep.

Stages 3 and 4 are deep sleep and together usually last around 40 minutes. These are the phases of sleep which are probably the most restorative. It is hard to wake a person in these stages, and if you do he will be disorientated and sluggish.

Stage 5 sleep is where dreaming occurs. It is also called rapid eye movement (REM) sleep, for obvious reasons. It is actually a higher level of arousal than levels 2, 3 and 4 sleep, involving increased heart and breathing rates, and the sleeper may sometimes wake up during this phase. If she does so suddenly, it can be frightening for her, as muscles are temporarily paralysed and this inability to move may persist for ten seconds or so after waking occurs. This most commonly happens out of a frightening dream (night terror), making the experience all the more disconcerting. REM sleep is probably when information which has been put to one side for one reason or another during the day is processed and organized emotionally.

The crucial point of Figure 2.1 is this: if you are over-aroused, your sleep pattern is the same as mine; it's just shifted upwards throughout the 24-hour cycle, because you are running too hot all the time. There is nothing especially wrong with your sleep; it's just reflecting your over-arousal. If you are afraid of not sleeping, you will be anxious (over-aroused) and it is obvious from this graph that you won't spend much time in the deeper, restorative stages.

The anatomy and physiology of sleep and circadian rhythms

Like any electrical device, which it is (just quite a complex one), the brain needs to be switched on in order to function. The switch is called the suprachiasmatic nucleus (SCN) and exists deep in the middle of the brain. It is switched on by light hitting the retina of the eye. By a circuitous route travelling via the upper spinal cord, it links with the pineal gland (Figure 2.2). This gland produces the hormone melatonin, the substance which turns on the sleep response by pushing arousal down. It is essentially our self-produced sedative. The SCN switches off production of melatonin by the pineal gland, thus switching the brain on into wakefulness. There is in fact a bit of a lag, with the rate of firing of the SCN being at its highest in the middle of the evening.

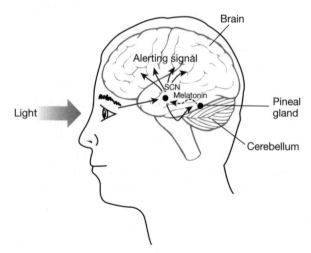

Figure 2.2 Brain structures involved in sleep

There are other factors which also affect the activity of the SCN, including the timing of meals, exercise, social activities and other routines, so that sleep patterns are not entirely dependent on light. Sleep–wake cycles are a product of all of the other regular routines and rhythms in our lives. This is our circadian rhythm.

Human beings have evolved to run on a 24-hour cycle, which is fortunate as that is how our world works. Not just sleep, but also body temperature and other metabolic functions vary depending on the time of day. All these functions are interrelated, so sleep rhythms are dependent on other body rhythms and vice versa. Our regular habits also affect our circadian rhythms. Interestingly, our internal body clock isn't perfect. If a human is deprived of a day–night cycle of light and dark for an extended period, she will naturally tend to fall into a circadian rhythm not of 24 hours, but nearer 25.

Opposing the SCN's tendency to switch off the pineal gland and thus to switch on the brain is the brain's natural drive to turn off when it has been awake for a long time. This physiological effect, known as the sleep load, builds through the waking day, so it is at its minimum first thing in the morning and its maximum last thing at night. As you sleep, the sleep load gradually falls, only to start rising again as soon as you wake up. This build-up of sleep load is mediated by a transmitter chemical (a chemical which allows nerve impulses to be passed from one nerve fibre to the next) in various parts of the brain, called GABA (gamma-aminobutyric acid). This is another of the brain's sedatives, though it works differently from melatonin, GABA being an electrical conductor between nerve fibres while melatonin is a hormone working through the blood supply to the SCN.

In the morning, the SCN is only beginning to get active, but as the sleep load is very low you wake up. In the evening, you stay awake despite a high and building sleep load because the SCN is very active. Only when the SCN starts to switch off a few hours after dark (that is, after darkness falls on the average length day) is the sleep load sufficiently unopposed to allow sleep (see Figure 2.3 overleaf). The other circadian rhythm routines keep the durations of sleep and wakefulness roughly constant through the year.

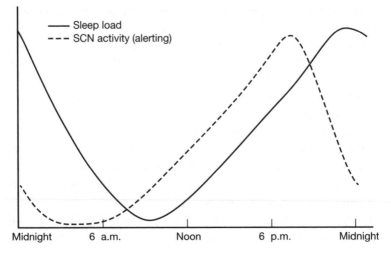

Figure 2.3 Sleep load and activity of SCN over 24 hours

Variation in sleep over time and in populations

Some people naturally need a lot of sleep and some a lot less. That is the same as for any characteristic which is distributed in a population on a continuum, such as height, IQ or strength, for example. When 'amount of sleep required' is plotted on a graph

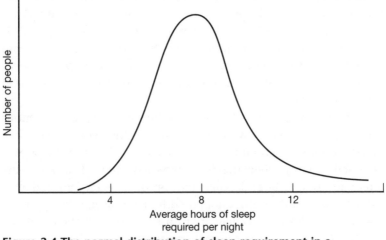

Figure 2.4 The normal distribution of sleep requirement in a population

for any population, with hours of sleep on one axis and number of people needing this amount of sleep on the other, the result, as for the other characteristics I mentioned, always forms the shape of a bell (Figure 2.4).

As you can see, most people need between 6.5 and 8.5 hours a night for optimal functioning, but a few people need ten hours a night and a few only five. If you are one of the people needing five hours, you may consider yourself a poor sleeper, but if that has always been how much you sleep, you aren't. That's just you.

As you get older, you need less sleep. A baby needs to sleep most of the time, a 15-year-old may sleep ten hours a night, but at 30 that's down to eight hours and at 70 to six hours. Again, the older person may assume she suffers from insomnia, whereas in fact six hours is all she needs (Figure 2.5).

Complicating this is the fact that young people tend to exhibit what is called phase delay: that is, left to their own devices, they tend to go to bed progressively later and get up later as well. Anyone who has had student offspring living with them during university vacations will know the struggle to get them out of bed before midday and the importance of buying them headphones to prevent the house being filled with heavy metal music at 2 a.m.

Conversely, older people exhibit phase advance, tending to move dinner and bedtime progressively earlier and being unable to sleep

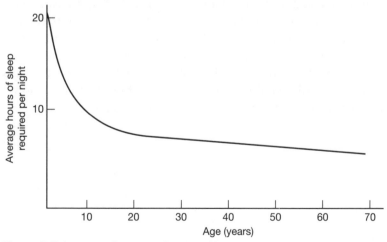

Figure 2.5 Average sleep requirement versus age

through to dawn. Waking at 5 a.m., they assume, often wrongly, that they are suffering from insomnia.

What all of this means for you

Understanding these principles of sleep is, in my view, quite important. It may be that you are sleeping more than you think, or that you don't in fact suffer from insomnia at all. If you do, it may be that it reflects wider issues which need to be addressed in your life, or it might be that some simple changes in your routine will do the trick.

There are, of course, a number of factors that can alter the normal pattern of sleep, which I will deal with in later chapters, but the bottom line is that if, for whatever reason, you don't spend much time in the deeper levels of sleep, you are unlikely to feel refreshed, and if REM sleep is reduced, you may have information-processing problems. If much of your sleep is in the lighter stages, you may even think that you aren't sleeping at all, because of partial awareness being present in stage 1 of sleep.

You need to do something about your high level of arousal throughout the day and particularly in the evening and night. This may mean doing something about your anxiety and attitudes about sleep.

You are going to need to look at your habits, helping your circadian rhythms to get in sync by searching for healthy routines. Most of all, you are going to need to be realistic in your aims and expectations about sleep, given your constitution and age.

I will come back to all of this later in the book. For now, it suffices to say that understanding how your sleep pattern naturally works is going to be an important factor in your sleeping better.

3

Why can't I sleep? I: General

So what is your sleep problem all about? How has it changed? When did it change? What was going on when it changed? Is the problem only during the working week? Is it difficulty going to sleep, waking too early in the morning, interrupted sleep or unrefreshing sleep? What are your habits and routines? What do you tend to do in the evenings? Do you consume caffeine? How much and at what time? Do you drink alcohol regularly? Why? Do you take any illicit drugs, particularly stimulant drugs, even occasionally? How are you generally? How is your mood? Is the stress you are under self-inflicted, at least in part? Do you have a way of relaxing? When do you get to sort out problems and planning? Do you take responsibility for everything and everyone and get overloaded? Do you worry a lot, particularly about the past and the future? Do you worry about not sleeping? What harm do you think will come from your insomnia? What have you done so far to try to deal with it? Do you exercise regularly, and at what time? What do you do when you've lain awake for a while without getting to sleep? What is your bedroom environment like? What medications are you on? Do you have a baby or older children, and if so how much do you do for them and what help do you get? Is there balance in your life? Do you take time for yourself? Are you resentful or angry much of the time? How much do you wish I would stop firing questions at you?

All right, I'll stop, but these are some of the questions which I would need to ask if I was assessing your sleep problem. As you can gather, there are a lot of factors which tend to add together to cause insomnia in most people. It's worth considering some of the main ones.

In my view, the key to managing most problems, including insomnia, is in understanding why it is happening to you and why now. So please bear with me through the long list of causes of insomnia in the next two chapters. Once you've worked out which causes apply to you, the solutions may well be obvious.

Stress

This is the single biggest cause of insomnia in the modern world. So many of us run at a million miles an hour and are stressed most of the time. For this reason I have given this subject a chapter of its own. If you can learn how to run at a lower level of arousal (see Chapter 2), there's a fair chance that your sleep will improve greatly.

There are effective ways of dealing with stress, but first of all you need to acknowledge that you are stressed, look for the reasons why, and change some things in your life which need to be and can be changed (see Chapter 8). The problem with the effective techniques for managing stress is that they are a complete waste of time to begin with – that is, until you become really good at them and they become second nature. This is why exactly the people who need these skills find it so hard to gain them. If you're overloaded and stressed, there isn't time to learn how not to be stressed.

More of this later. For now, I will simply lay this marker: *you're probably going to need to give time you don't think you have to dealing with your stress levels if you are going to succeed in your attempt to sleep better.*

Habits and routines

As I explained in Chapter 2, your body runs on rhythms. These in turn are set by external cues. The more regular these are, the greater the chance of your body routinely following a predictable and regular sleep–wake cycle. Given that the length of daytime and night-time varies so much at high latitudes such as in the UK, our sleep–wake cycle relies greatly on the habits which drive our circadian rhythms. Our SCN wakefulness switch (see Chapter 2) needs a cue to switch off so that levels of our sleep hormone, melatonin, can rise, turning off wakefulness and inducing sleep. In the absence of a day of constant length, which we don't have in the UK, this cue is provided by our regular routines.

Having a life in which you eat, work, exercise, socialize, study, sleep or rest at different and unpredictable times each day makes it difficult for your body to get into a rhythm compatible with good sleep.

Your body needs time to prepare for sleep. While eating and exercising are routines which help you to sleep well, they shouldn't be engaged in too near bedtime, as doing so within two or three hours of the time you hope to sleep may disrupt your sleep cycle.

It isn't just the regular timing of your routines, but also what they entail. I once had a patient whose insomnia at first glance appeared difficult to understand. He ate healthily at regular times, not too near bedtime, did the same with exercise, avoided tea, coffee and alcohol in the evening and spent a good hour reading before turning the lights off. It all sounded ideal. Then I asked him what he read at bedtime. It turned out his reading material was the *Financial Times* and world stock market reports. He was a stockbroker who wanted to be ahead of the game for when the markets opened early next morning. Obviously, he was totally switched on at bedtime; this is incompatible with sleep. To him, the concept of reading something pointless and unrelated to potential profit was anathema. Because he couldn't get to sleep, he had difficulty getting up in the morning, so he was resistant to the idea of rising early to study what he needed to.

To sleep well, you need to learn how to waste time regularly, to be boringly predictable and to tolerate the idea that things may not go your way in the short term if you do what is needed to achieve the good sleep you desire in the longer term.

Balance

Everything in life is about balance. Not just work–life balance, though it is important to achieve that, but balance in everything else too. This means achieving a balance between your family's needs and your own, socializing versus quiet time, exercise versus rest, using your mind versus blobbing in front of the TV, and so on. The list is endless.

The point is that if your life is out of balance, with you going hell for leather after only one goal, you are going to run too hot and lack the cues which your body needs to switch on the sleep response. You can't expect your body to provide you with regular rhythms such as consistent sleep when you aren't providing it with balanced rhythms to work on and are running at a white hot level of arousal.

Children and partners

I don't know about you, but I find babies wind me up. Their cry sounds to me like it comes straight from the pit of hell. I guess it's because I haven't got female hormones to help me, though I know many men seem to enjoy at least their own infants. Even if you do, there is no denying that they aren't good for sleep. The interrupted nights caused by a baby's variably timed nocturnal crying can disrupt your sleep pattern considerably beyond the time when your child sleeps through to morning.

I hear many of my patients – and I remember it myself – complaining that, as their children get older, their demands only increase. Evenings and weekends are taken up providing a taxi service, once you've finished doing their washing, cooking their food and helping with their homework.

Where's the wind-down time? The answer is that there isn't any unless you sometimes say no, demand they pull their weight with the chores and include yourself in the equation when everybody's needs and wishes are being worked out.

Then there's your spouse or partner. While you love him to bits, he expects you to do pretty much everything at home while he watches the football. Then, when you finally collapse in a heap into bed, he snores so loudly that you'd need a general anaesthetic or to have your auditory apparatus surgically removed in order to get a wink of sleep.

All right, there's a bit of sexual stereotyping here, but I do find that more women than men complain of being taken advantage of in terms of allocation of domestic duties and of their partner snoring. I suspect that the latter is because male alcohol consumption is on average higher than that of their female partners. Obesity, the other main precipitant of snoring, is spread more evenly between the sexes.

Sleep behaviour and environment

The bedroom has only two purposes, sleep and, in some circum-stances, sex. While this book isn't a sex manual, it is worth pointing out that (only on average; there are exceptions) men tend to be sleepier after sex, whereas many women feel more awake. It may be appropriate to negotiate with your partner about timing of sexual intercourse, taking this into account. This may need some diplo-macy. Utterances such as 'Well, how's about it then, 'cos I could do with a good sleep' are unlikely to elicit the desired response.

Regularly reading for 20 minutes or so before turning the light off can be helpful, but your reading material needs to be chosen care-fully (see page 63). Complex text, exciting thrillers, horror novels or racy romps are counter-productive, heightening rather than lowering arousal. I will advise on appropriate reading material later on. While many of us read from our tablets or back-lit Kindles, this isn't ideal either. There is evidence that the blue light from LCD and computer screens can confuse the normal circadian sleep–wake response in some particularly light-sensitive individuals.

The most destructive screen in the bedroom for sleeping is the TV. Not only does the light confuse the sleep pathway described in Chapter 2, but the TV engages the brain (yes, I know, it rots the brain as well), and the association between bed and brain-engage-ment trains you to stay awake. While I can't think of anything more tedious than *Keeping Up with the Kardashians*, one of my wife's current favourites, it isn't soporific for me. It is for her, so this is one show which she watches alone. Anything which annoys you will tend to keep you awake, while anything comfortably familiar will prepare you for sleep.

Many people who suffer from insomnia take naps during the day. While this is completely understandable, it only serves to ensure poor sleep the following night, as sleep need is spread over 24 hours. Any sleep taken during the day will be subtracted from the time you will be expected to sleep the next night. It also makes it harder to achieve the circadian rhythm of which the sleep–wake cycle is a part.

Light

I have touched on this above, relating to computer and TV screens. It is worth emphasizing, though, that light is a crucial cue for circadian rhythms. Bright light near bedtime hinders the gradual fall of arousal which leads to sleep. Long, light evenings in high latitude summers can delay sleep onset if not managed properly. Curtains may need to be drawn before dusk. If you have to work late, doing so under bright strip-lighting is very likely to cause difficulty getting to sleep. Even your digital alarm clock can be a factor, if the display is bright. Most such devices have a dimmer setting.

Expectations

So many of my patients have unrealistic and self-defeating expectations about their sleep pattern. However tense and wound up, depressed, sick, inactive or loaded up with stimulants they may be, they demand of their sleep that it should always deliver a high-quality eight hours, *particularly tonight* as it's so important that I'm in top shape tomorrow. Come on, give me a break – it isn't going to happen. Acceptance of this fact is, for most of us, very difficult. Your sleep is likely to be on its worst behaviour when you most need it to cooperate. I'm sorry, but that's just the way it is.

Que sera sera is difficult for doers and shakers. On this one, though, acceptance that you can't make it happen is the key.

Thinking pattern

Following hot on the heels of the unrealistic expectations described above are catastrophic thoughts. 'If I don't sleep well tonight, it'll be a disaster.' Are you sure? Yes? Then you will make your own prediction come true (see the Introduction). Many of my patients have very catastrophic thinking and assumptions about the consequences of poor sleep. These have little basis in evidence. The truth is that you can get by without much sleep for one or two nights, though it isn't ideal. It is, as I have said before, the worry about the consequences of not sleeping which causes the disablement you associate with the last time you slept poorly. Catastrophic thinking stops you sleeping well.

There are a number of other characteristic thinking patterns which lead a person to suffer from anxiety or depression, both of which interfere with sleep (see Chapter 4) and which tend to be associated with unhelpful behaviours. For example, selective abstraction refers to a person considering only those aspects and events which back up his negative view of himself, the world or the future. So he says to himself, 'I've got to sleep well, because in the past, when I've slept badly, everything has gone wrong.' He has abstracted from his memories a time ten years ago when he did badly in an exam, having slept fitfully the previous night. He is forgetting that he hadn't revised properly for the exam, having suffered with flu for the preceding fortnight, and that he slept equally poorly before all his other exams, in which he ended up doing well. He also uses generalization, telling himself, 'Because I once performed badly after a disturbed night's sleep, I will always always fail when I don't sleep well.'

As a result of these unhelpful thinking patterns, he gets very anxious prior to bedtime, drinks a lot of alcohol to help him sleep and goes to bed unusually early. These thoughts, emotions and behaviours are the main causes of his poor sleep.

Identifying these problematic thoughts and compensatory actions are the basis of cognitive behavioural therapy (CBT), a much-used therapeutic strategy for insomnia (see Chapter 9).

Psychodynamics

This refers to the things we learnt as kids, literally what makes your mind run. A child is a blank computer disc and childhood is about programming the computer. If we learn some stuff (are educated), learn a moral sense so as not to get into too much trouble, learn 'I'm OK' and 'The world's OK', we tend to get a reasonably happy and carefree life, because we assume things will turn out all right in the end, and in any case it's not our fault if it doesn't. If we don't get this programming as kids, we're all right if the world smiles on us, but if the world turns hostile we tend to try too hard to fix it.

The phenomenon which is particularly relevant in the context of sleep is resonance. This means that we are specially vulnerable to things which remind us of events or circumstances that traumatized us in the past. If bedtime was a time of fear when you were a child, because of emotional, physical or sexual abuse, or because of other circumstances which as a child you linked with bed, such as parental rows, bedwetting or myriad other negative experiences, you learnt to be fearful at this time. When something comes up now to trigger that emotional memory, you're likely to experience fear at bedtime and difficulty sleeping as a result.

Feelings and planning

Life gets very full. There just isn't time to fit everything in. The only time we really get to review the day and how we feel about it is bedtime. At night, things tend to get out of perspective, magnified. So reverses take on a blacker hue, perceived insults and hurts get ruminated upon, unfairnesses resented. All of this churns around your head and stops you sleeping. You tend to fantasize either about the catastrophe to which it will all lead or about what you will do tomorrow to put the architect of your misfortune and humiliation in his place.

The thing is that, in the entire history of humanity, nobody has ever carried these fantasies through, thank goodness, so they are a complete waste of time. All they achieve is to wind you up and to stop you sleeping. Fear, worry, anger and resentment are all really the same thing and are experienced by the body as a high state of arousal.

In this space after lights out, other random thoughts also pop into your head. 'I mustn't forget to buy the cat food tomorrow.' 'I wonder if Bill will call tomorrow, maybe I should call him.' 'What shall I get Auntie Nora for her birthday?' You try to shut these thoughts out, but the computer that is your brain has a pop-up mechanism which keeps inserting them back into your consciousness. It doesn't believe that you will sort these issues out any other time, as you don't have any, so it keeps reminding you. You can't shut down a computer and keep it running. Your brain stays awake while it's thinking and planning.

Substances

Alcohol is our favourite drug. Yes, it is a drug and not a very good one at that. The main problem is that it reverses its own effect, both immediately and over time.

When you have a drink it calms you. When you have several, it puts you to sleep. But when it wears off, you get an equal and opposite effect, feeling more anxious and waking early in an agitated state. In addition, the normal architecture of sleep (see Chapter 2) is disrupted, and much less of your sleep is in the deeper, restorative stages 3 and 4. Then, even after modest amounts of alcohol, measured anxiety levels the day after evening drinking are higher than in people who have abstained. So much for taking a couple of drinks to help you sleep before an important day ahead.

That is the immediate effect of alcohol. The longer-term effects of regular heavy drinking on sleep are worse still, particularly on getting to sleep. The reversal effect means that, while having a couple of drinks gets you to sleep quicker initially, in the long term when done regularly it makes getting to sleep a much longer process. Then, when you stop drinking, it becomes even harder. That is alcohol withdrawal and it can happen at much lower levels of regular alcohol consumption than you would think (though a small drink a few times a week isn't a problem).

I'm not suggesting getting dependent on tranquillizers or sleeping tablets, but they are better than alcohol. There is only one safe use for alcohol and that is occasional social recreation. Using it to help you sleep always leads to problems. Don't take a nightcap.

Caffeine is also a drug. It is related to amphetamine, being a stimulant, albeit a weaker one. It has a long half-life (the time it takes for the level in your blood stream to fall from its peak level to a half of that), around six hours, meaning that there's still a quarter of it in your system 12 hours after that strong cup of coffee. It's best, therefore, to avoid caffeinated coffee, tea, Red Bull or cola from the afternoon on. Interesting, then, that tea has so often been consumed in the late afternoon that the light meal taken at that time of day has been named after it. Many a dinner party ends with coffee and chocolates (chocolate is also mildly stimulant, the cocoa bean and coffee bean being related). While some good sleepers may get away with this, poor sleepers won't. Also beware of caffeine in health drinks and medicines. Many proprietary brands of cold medicines or paracetamol contain it in significant quantities.

I'm not going to talk a lot about illicit drugs here. Suffice it to say that most of them can interfere seriously with sleep. Amphetamine ('speed'), cocaine ('coke'), ecstasy ('E') and most designer drugs are strong stimulants. Sedative drugs such as heroin, tranquillizers (downers) and even cannabis will initially induce sleep, but over time will wreck it because, like all addictive drugs, they reverse their own effect over time with regular use.

I will write more about sleeping tablets later (see Chapter 11). They also have the potential to lead to addiction and to reverse their effect in the long term, though some are worse than others. Overall, I have to say that I have seen more harm than good come from long-term use of these drugs. Remember, a tranquillizer at higher dosage becomes a sleeping tablet (there may be exceptions to this, which I will discuss in Chapter 11), so if tranquillizers are addictive, sleeping tablets will be more so.

Hormones

Hormones regulate pretty much everything in the body. I have already outlined how the hormone melatonin regulates sleep, but there are several others which also have an effect, including the stress hormones adrenaline and cortisol, which I will discuss in Chapter 4.

The fact that women complain of sleep problems more often than men is in no small part caused by fluctuations in the hormones progesterone and oestrogen, which control the menstrual cycle. Progesterone is a calming, sedative hormone. Its level in the blood stream falls quite rapidly in the few days before the start of your menstrual period. The rapidity of this fall and the degree of your sensitivity to the level of progesterone varies between women. Those most affected experience very disturbed sleep in the premenstrual period, with sleep being much improved within a day or two of the onset of their period.

Many women also experience insomnia around the time of the menopause and for some time afterwards. This appears to be caused more by a fall in the production of oestrogen, though falling pro-gesterone levels may also be a factor.

As men get older, production of the male hormone testosterone falls (to a lesser extent the same is true for women, who also produce this hormone, in smaller quantities). There does seem to be a link between this fall and poor sleep in some men, though the mechanism isn't entirely clear. It may be that falling testosterone levels lead to reduced motivation and activity, this in turn reducing the sleep load (see Chapter 2).

Anybody with an overactive thyroid gland (thyrotoxicosis) is likely to have difficulty sleeping. Thyroxine (thyroid hormone) sets the body's metabolic rate. If metabolism is set too high, the low arousal levels needed for sleep are difficult to achieve. Conversely, those with thyroid under-activity (myxoedema) may become list-less and passive, again reducing sleep load and leading to insomnia. You just can't win with hormones.

Fitness and general health

As I have explained, regular activity is important for sleep. The less physically fit you are, the less likely you are to be physically active (this works both ways). Obesity is linked to breathing problems and sleep apnoea (see p. 87). There is a vicious cycle here, with poor sleep exacerbating health problems, which in turn impair sleep. People with chronic illnesses tend to put insomnia near the top of their list of problems. It's a difficult one, as many people in poor health cannot be physically active. While this means that they don't need as much sleep as those engaged in vigorous physical exertion, that is little comfort when lying awake with your symp-toms in the early hours.

I'll look at how physical and mental illnesses interfere with sleep next.

4

Why can't I sleep? II: Illnesses and their treatment

Most illnesses, both physical and mental, cause poor sleep, directly as a symptom, as a result of pain or discomfort or sometimes resulting from treatment.

Physical illnesses

Illnesses are scary, some very much so. Fear is a state of high arousal and as such is the opposite of sleep. Unfortunately, my profession is often to blame here. In the absence of good information from your doctor on the likely course and prognosis of your condition, you'll tend to turn to the internet, in which exaggeration, scare stories and nightmares abound.

Many of my patients trace the start of their insomnia to a stay in hospital. Don't get me wrong; I'm not criticizing NHS staff, who do their best with scant resources, but if I'm really bad for the rest of my life I know where I'll spend eternity. Hell is the medical assessment ward of my local district general hospital. The constant alarms from cardiac monitors which are ignored by the staff (what's the point in an alarm if nothing is done when it goes off?), punctuated by occasional shouts from the confused man in the corner, the lack of any sense of what to expect next, the boredom, the humiliation of having to call for a bedpan and the ferocious admonition which results if you try to go to the loo . . . all these add up to an environment of wakeful fear and misery which tends to persist when you go home. An episode of serious physical illness leaves you feeling vulnerable, fearful and hyper-vigilant. Your circadian rhythm ceases to work, having been deprived of the routines of your everyday life. Stress and fear, the constant bedfellows of serious physical illness, lead to a rise in circulating adrenaline and cortisol levels, further disrupting your circadian rhythm and your ability to develop the drowsiness needed to get to sleep.

Pain is a feature of many illnesses and is never a good thing, but can often be coped with during the day. The hustle and bustle of life forces your attention away from discomfort. But when the lights go off, there's nothing to distract you and pain takes centre stage. Many people are in pain all the time; it's a wonder they can sleep at all. In addition, pain limits your ability to take exercise, which, as I have outlined, is an important factor in promoting sleep. Insomnia, I'm reliably informed, is one of the worst aspects of arthritis. Those with cancer say the same thing.

There is no division between mind and body. Physical illnesses all affect your mind and mental illnesses your body. If you're tense and anxious much of the time, you may develop a stomach ulcer from the production of too much stomach acid. The ulcer isn't 'all in your mind'; it's a hole in your stomach. Or you may get high blood pressure. That isn't imaginary; it can be potentially very dangerous. Physical illness leads to stress, which leads to more illness, and both contribute to difficulty sleeping.

Heart disease, with the fear it causes, is particularly associated with insomnia, as are respiratory diseases such as bronchitis, emphysema and asthma. Hypoxia (lack of oxygen in the blood stream), which those with chronic respiratory diseases get used to over time, disrupts the normal sleep–wake cycle. Bowel problems often present with complaints of insomnia. Abdominal pain, discomfort and bloating, constipation and diarrhoea are all closely linked with stress and poor sleep. Irritable bowel syndrome (IBS), which involves all of these symptoms, is experienced most often by people who tend to anxiety. Whether it is the underlying anxiety or the very unpleasant bowel symptoms, which are often at their worst through the night, those with IBS often experience poor sleep. Bladder and prostate problems may lead to several trips to the toilet each night, making normal sleep architecture impossible.

Hormones and sleep are inextricably linked, as I've already mentioned. Many diabetics sleep poorly and improving sleep is an important factor in improving control of blood sugar.

Enough, I think, of this list of physical illnesses for which insomnia is a problem. The truth is that most people with severe, painful, debilitating or chronic physical illnesses sleep poorly. It is a major part of their suffering.

Many people with chronic pain are on regular analgesics. The most commonly used are the non-steroidal anti-inflammatory drugs (NSAIDs) such as aspirin, ibuprofen, naproxen and diclofenac. These tablets tend to upset the stomach, which can impair sleep. Worse are the opiate analgesics, such as codeine, dihydrocodeine, tramadol and morphine. These drugs act on the brain and, among their other actions, are tranquillizing and sleep inducing. They are addictive and, like all addictive drugs, reverse their own effect with long-term use, thus impairing sleep. Then, when they are stopped, particularly when this is done quickly, sleep gets even worse (a withdrawal effect). Top of the list of sleep-wrecking analgesics is alcohol, often used dependently by those in chronic pain. The single most effective measure which could be taken to reduce the burden both of chronic pain and sleeplessness in the population would be to ban alcohol. Don't worry, it'll never happen. Too many politicians rely upon it.

Mental illnesses

While insomnia is a feature of most psychological conditions, it is mood disorders and anxiety states for which it tends to be the biggest problem, the worst being stress-related depression.

In bipolar disorder (manic depressive illness), mood fluctuates between depression and elation. At both extremes sleep is reduced. During a manic phase, people may not sleep for days, and if they do, sleep is brief and fitful. During the depressed phase the sleep loss is the same as in ordinary (unipolar) depression.

Anxiety disorders tend to lead to initial insomnia: that is, difficulty getting to sleep is the main problem, mainly because anxious rumination makes it impossible to enter the relaxed state needed to trigger the sleep response. Typically, an anxious person can sleep a fair number of hours once she gets to sleep, if there is sufficient time left in the night to do so, though sleep may be shallow and unrefreshing because arousal never falls sufficiently to enter stages 3 and 4 of sleep. Dreams may be vivid and frightening. As outlined above, the high circulating levels of adrenaline and cortisol which occur in anxiety states are another important factor.

People with anxiety often get dependent on benzodiazepine tranquillizers such as diazepam (Valium) or lorazepam (Ativan) and sleeping tablets acting on the same receptors (see below). These are addictive drugs which cause immediate relief from anxiety and insomnia (which is an understandably compelling reason to keep taking them) but inevitably cause a reverse of their own effect over time with constant use, thus wrecking sleep and exacerbating anxiety. There is a very long history, covering several millennia, of new drugs coming along with the promise of a non-addictive solution to anxiety, only in due course to be found to be addictive. Don't believe anyone who tells you that a new drug gives instant relief from anxiety without any risk of addiction. Drugs such as the SSRI antidepressants, on the contrary, lead to a slow reduction in anxiety over several weeks. This delay in action makes their capacity to cause addiction very low.

In depressive illness (clinical depression, major depressive disorder), the typical disturbance, on the contrary, is early morning waking. The person falls asleep easily enough, only to wake in the early hours, often being unable to fall back to sleep. The hours before dawn can be particularly horrible owing to diurnal variation of mood: that is, someone feeling at his worst when he wakes up and gradually better as the day goes on.

The other typical symptoms of depressive illness are: depressed mood (obviously) and a series of 'loss ofs' – that is, loss of appetite and weight (these conversely may be increased), energy, enthusiasm, concentration, memory, confidence, self-esteem, sex drive, drive, enjoyment, patience, feelings, optimism: loss of just about anything and everything. If you're experiencing most of these symptoms, you may be sleeping poorly because you have a depressive illness. That's actually good news, as it usually isn't difficult to treat.

In practice, anxiety and depression often go together, so many people get sandwiched between the double whammy of initial insomnia and early morning waking.

There is an interrelationship between sleep disturbance and depression which is, as yet, unclear. It used to be assumed that sleep loss was a symptom of depressive illness, but there is now an increasingly popular theory that it may in fact be the cause. This theory points out that the hormonal disturbance found in major depression (particularly very high levels of cortisol) is the same as found in hibernating animals. It's strange that lower primates respond to a rise in cortisol levels by falling asleep, while we get depressed and can't sleep. This is probably because of our large and complex brains. The sleep load needed to switch off the waking signal described in Chapter 2 probably doesn't build as it should, or the body fails to recognize it, in the presence of high levels of cortisol. Remember, this stress hormone is produced by the body in response to extended perceived threat. It wouldn't work well if you fell asleep while being chased by a sabre-toothed tiger.

In any case, early morning waking is one of the most distressing symptoms of depressive illness and can often persist for some time after the other symptoms of the condition have settled. One of the main reasons is that, in some people, the drugs most often used to treat the illness can interfere with sleep. The SSRI anti-depressants, such as fluoxetine (Prozac), citalopram (Cipramil), escitalopram (Cipralex) and sertraline (Lustral) all quite commonly cause vivid dreaming. People may wake during such dreams and, if they are nightmares, may be fearful, leading to difficulty getting back to sleep. Other, more sedative antidepressants such as mir-

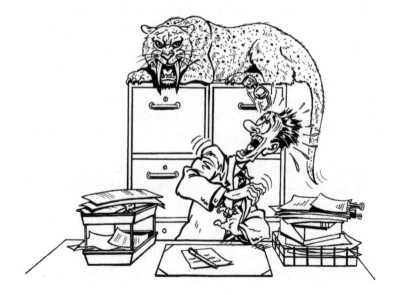

tazapine (Zispin) and the older tricyclic drugs such as amitriptyline (Triptizol) may promote sleep, but what isn't clear is whether they may compromise its quality (less time in the deep phases of sleep). There isn't any good evidence of sedative antidepressants being addictive, meaning that they don't, as far as we know, reverse their own effects over time.

The same can't be said for benzodiazepine hypnotics such as temazepam or the z-drugs, zaleplon, zolpidem and zopiclone, which act on the same receptors in the brain. While the addictive potential of zopiclone in particular is quite low, all drugs of this kind can cause dependence and, in the long term, may make your sleep worse if used regularly for extended periods. As I will mention later, this needs to be kept in proportion. If you have been on a z-drug for years at a steady low dosage, don't suddenly come off it without talking to your GP first.

Over-the-counter hypnotics are mainly sedative antihistamines, which have a low addictive potential. Sensibly, though, the manufacturers discourage long-term regular use.

Drugs really aren't a good long-term solution to insomnia and many will make the problem worse in the long run. Understand the cause(s) of the problem and deal with them if this is at all possible. This will not only provide enduring improvement in your sleep, but will lead to you enjoying better health too.

5

Why am I over-aroused?

Over-arousal is the commonest cause of insomnia. It means that you are too stressed, tense, alert, excited or however else you experience your body physiology running too hot.

Stress is actually a misnomer when used in this context. What we really mean is strain. These are engineering terms. Stress is the load put on a structure. Strain is what happens when the load either exceeds the tolerance of the structure or when the stress is applied in a direction or manner for which the structure isn't designed. So a suspension bridge can take heavy lorries rumbling over it every day, but when wind of a particular speed from a particular direction is applied to it for too long, it collapses.

Human beings can cope with an amazing amount, so long as the demands are the ones they are designed for. In this, as in so much else in life, everyone is different. One of my best friends at medical school loved the drama and crisis of medical emergencies. She was never happier than when up to her elbows in blood and guts, but got bored if an issue dragged into the next day. I hate crises; I find them annoying, worrying and stultifying. But give me a knotty problem which takes months or years to resolve and I'm in my element. What she enjoyed, I found stressful, and vice versa. Happily, she became a surgeon and I went into psychiatry, both of us being well suited to our occupations.

Having said all of this, most people talk about being stressed, so this is the term which I will use, risking the wrath of any literary pedants among you.

If you are stressed for much of the time, you are either overloaded or facing demands for which you are ill suited. Some situations are very stressful for almost everyone, where there is no obvious way out from the stress. Some people and places are also stressful to most people. However, more often, *stress doesn't make you stressed, or ill: you do.*

It's worth asking yourself a few questions about your stress. Is my stress really unavoidable, or am I choosing it? What are the 'givens' which keep me in this situation? Is this stressful person who I call a friend really a friend? Can I reduce the stress which this place causes me? Do I have to stay here?

Causes of stress can be separated out into those which are mainly external (stressful situations, people and places) and mainly internal (ways of thinking and operating which bring stress upon you).

External causes of stress

There's no doubt that life is more stressful than it once was. The main reason is that the demands on us keep changing all the time. This is natural, because we have to adapt to an ever-changing world. But what politicians and some business leaders fail to appreciate is that change is an injury. It makes people stressed and less good at what they do. Pace of change needs to be managed carefully. The trouble is that this goes against human nature and in particular the nature of our leaders. Politicians are like dogs. Put them on a new patch and they feel compelled metaphorically to urinate around the perimeter, just to show that it is theirs. They change everything in their own image, only for the new lot to change it all back again. It was always thus. In AD 66 Caius Petronius, a Roman commander, complained that his bosses were demoralizing and demotivating his troops by insisting on changes in order to persuade the populace that progress was being achieved.

Our bosses don't let us learn through our mistakes any more. Society has become increasingly punitive. As soon as a disaster occurs, the hunt is on for someone to blame, under the pretext of 'accountability'. This is a shame, as that wasn't what the term was coined for. It was actually developed in the USA several decades ago as, at the time, a radical new way of doing business. Instead of the boss telling his minions what to do and them passing on instructions to those below them, whole areas of responsibility were devolved downwards. Those at the bottom of the business were expected to learn on the job, including learning from their mistakes. These errors were not to be punished, but to be learnt from. Thus the workforce gained expertise and were empowered. Typically, in our sado-masochistic culture, we have taken this excellent concept and turned it into a way of making people feel frightened. Failure is punished. If people succeed, we simply increase our demands upon them until they fail. Ever-increasing demands with ever-diminishing resources and influence is a common lament in my consulting room.

One stress or demand isn't usually a problem. It's when several demands are conflicting that we get into difficulties. There are your needs (emotional and physical), those of your employer, your family, your friends, the Inland Revenue and many others. There simply isn't the time or resources to satisfy them all. You can't keep everyone happy all the time. Most of my patients deal with this insoluble equation by ignoring their own needs completely. It can't last, though, as too much stress for too long leads to illness.

Some people are toxic. If you spend enough time with them, you'll suffer from stress. There isn't sufficient space to describe them all here, but you'll find them in my book *Stress-Related Illness* (Sheldon Press, 2007). There's not a lot you can do with these people as they are better at being toxic than you are at resisting them; they've been doing it all their lives. The trick is in identifying them and avoiding them.

Equally, some places are toxic. If you work in an environment which runs on fear, manipulation and bullying, you'll suffer from stress unless you're a cynical opportunist. They love toxic environments, as these places offer opportunities to employ their manipulative skills to advantage, in the moral vacuum created by weak or toxic leadership. If you're not one of those you're going to struggle, because the organization isn't about to change into a nurturing meritocracy just because you say so.

We learn to be stressed as children. If our parents, teachers and peers fail to teach us that 'I'm OK and the world is OK', we tend to lead our lives fearfully, expecting the worst and constantly guarding against it. If our parents really mess up on a frequent basis, we can develop learned helplessness. If you aren't taught that when you do good things good things happen, or that when you do nothing or bad things the result is bad, you learn instead that 'It doesn't matter what I do or don't do, I'm powerless to affect the world. I might as well give up.' Life is stressful and depressing for a person who learns

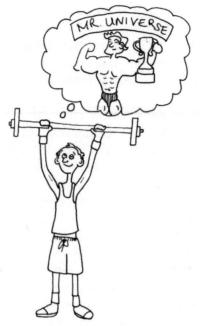

Cognitive dissonance

through childhood to be helpless. As described in Chapter 3, we get particularly stressed by things which remind us of, or resonate with, things which caused us stress or distress during our formative years.

You need to be realistic. The little guy in the cartoon is pumping weights, thinking that if he trains enough, he'll become Mr Universe and all the girls will admire him. No you won't, because you're a scrawny little runt. At best, you'll strain a muscle. But look, you're a great guy with a terrific sense of humour and loads of talents. Play to your strengths, not to your limitations. Cognitive dissonance is the distance between your ideal self and your real self. If your cognitive dissonance is large, you're going to be stressed and disappointed much of the time.

Internal causes of stress

We usually think of people suffering from stress as weak. In fact, the opposite is usually true. They tend to be those who do too much, expect too much of themselves and put everyone else's needs before their own. They hate letting people down and need to keep everyone happy all the time. They have a strong conscience and sense of responsibility. They avoid risk, because they can't allow themselves to fail. They are competitive and striving. They have broad shoulders and a safe pair of hands, but they are sensitive and easily hurt by criticism.

Stress is caused by spending too much time in the past or the future. The author Eckhart Tolle, who wrote the book *The Power of Now*, points out that it is impossible to be happy unless you are able to be fully present, now, to experience the present moment. Equally, it is very difficult to be unhappy if you are here, experiencing only the present. I suppose that if you are trapped in a cupboard with a rabid dog you won't be too chipper, but in most ordinary life situations, being present means being content. In any case, our takes on the past and the future are myths, the past being tainted by our selective recollection and interpretation and the future by our fear and catastrophization. What you worry about doesn't happen, though something else does. The only reality we possess is now.

Our attempts to control life cause a lot of our stress. You can't control life, not really. Trying to nail it down is like trying to nail down an armful of eels; you'll just make a mess and hurt yourself. By all means do what you can, put some preparation in, but as John Lennon famously said, 'Life is what happens while you're making other plans.' As a friend once advised me: 'Don't walk or run down escalators in underground stations. As likely as not, if you do, the tube train will have just left when you get to the bottom.'

To continue the plagiarism theme, the American pop TV psychologist 'Dr Phil' holds that much stress in relationships and marriages is caused by 'right-fighting'. This means that couples often deal with their differing needs and perspectives by fighting over who is right. They both state and restate their views over and over again, ever louder, under the mistaken belief that eventually their perspective will prevail. No it won't, because neither of you is either right or wrong. You're arguing over feelings and experiences, not facts. Because you know each other's weak points really well, when the discussion degenerates into mutual recrimination you are both able to deliver the really hurtful killer blow. There's an unnecessary internal cause of stress, right there.

Value judgements, such as good, bad, admirable, pathetic, beautiful, ugly, interesting, boring, and so on, don't tell you anything about the world, just about the values of the person making the judgement. Stressed people tend to be full of these judgements, particularly about themselves.

You are responsible for finding balance in your life. Not just work–life balance, but also balance between your needs and those of others, exercise versus rest, doing useful things versus blobbing in front of the TV. Stress results from a lack of balance in your life. It is our givens that prevent us from finding this balance. If it is given that you must have your large house, your big car and private medical insurance and that your kids must be privately educated, you're going to spend much of your life miserable and stressed, unless you're very lucky or talented. If you are an unemployed single mother of three children under the age of 5 with no support, it's impossible to be a perfect mum. If it's a given that you must be, you'll get stressed and probably ill, which certainly isn't in your kids' interests. It isn't necessary anyway, as research on child-rearing shows that being 'good enough' as a parent is better for your kids than being perfect. These are just two examples; there are a thousand other givens which lead to stress. Stressed people don't challenge their givens, they assume them.

I've already talked about the importance of moderating alcohol consumption and taking regular exercise for sleep. These are also, of course, major factors in worsening or moderating stress.

This has been a very quick trip through the causes of stress, which leads to the over-arousal which in turn lies behind insomnia in most people. If you can manage to get control over your stress, your sleep will improve. I will deal with how to achieve this later (see Chapters 8 and 9). There's more detail if you need it in *Stress-Related Illness*. For now, a final word on stress: a sports psychologist, Dr Bob Rotella, wrote a very successful book entitled *Golf is not a Game of Perfect*.

Life isn't a game of perfect either.

6

Some other problems which interfere with sleep

Jet lag

I'm married to an American and cross the pond quite often. I'm now familiar with the odd feeling I get for the first few days over there and after returning. At first I thought I was getting anxious and depressed, with malaise, irritability and sleep disturbance, which was strange as I love the States, but now I realize that it's just jet lag and I wait for it to pass, as it always does in a few days. I know than my melatonin secretion is temporarily on the blink and my cortisol levels a tad too high, but that they will right themselves in time.

For pilots, cabin crew and business people whose responsibilities are worldwide, it's difficult to be so phlegmatic, as much of their working lives can be spent in this state. I actually get it worse after east to west travel, but it's much commoner to experience more severe symptoms flying west to east. The conventional explanation for this is that, with the body's natural circadian rhythm being on a cycle of between 24 and 25 hours, a time change involving a longer day involves less of a challenge than one making the day shorter. I don't actually buy this, as the odd half an hour here or there doesn't really make much difference to the nervous system. I think it's much more likely to be due to us finding it difficult to go to sleep early, whereas we can take a nap in the middle of the day after lunch when we know we have an elongated day ahead, without disrupting our circadian rhythm very much.

In any case, jet lag can disrupt sleep well beyond the duration of other symptoms (typically around a day of symptoms for every time zone crossed). This is because sleep follows a habitual pattern. We all know that once we start waking up at 3.17 a.m. we keep doing so for several nights running. If typically your least deep sleep occurs at around this time, all you need to wake up then is to be a bit more aroused than normal. Jet lag, involving anxiety as it often does, makes such interrupted sleep more frequent. If you get anxious about your interrupted sleep when you wake up in the early hours, the anxiety stops you going back to sleep and makes it more likely that such awakening will occur the next night, and so on. Conversely, if you don't worry about the temporary disruption in your sleep, instead waiting patiently for normal sleep to return, the body's normal circadian rhythm will be restored soon enough, because it responds to the light and your daily habits in your new location.

Shift work

When a service needs to run 24 hours a day, somebody has to work the night shift. This inevitably causes sleep problems for many. The issue is at its worst during and just after each change in shift. It would be better for your sleep if you stayed permanently on one shift or another, even if it is the night shift, except that you want to have a life at weekends. Your partner, kids and friends are around and doing stuff during the day and you want to join them. Working nights, you therefore go through a more or less 12-hour phase shift twice a week. Then when your work hours flip again it's all change once more. Your body isn't well designed for this, running as it does on a regular circadian rhythm.

In addition, there is the problem of light. As I explained in Chapter 2, sleep cycles rely on a regular 24-hour pattern of rising and falling intensity of full spectrum light (not the yellow light of light bulbs). Trying to wake up and function when it is dark and to sleep after a drive home in daylight goes against your body's natural rhythm, particularly in winter (in summer we get used to going to bed when it's not completely dark anyway). Your melatonin levels and your SCN wakefulness switch are working in the wrong direction.

It's not surprising, therefore, that shift workers often experience insomnia.

Restless leg syndrome

This very unpleasant condition, which tends to run in families, affects up to 10 per cent of the population, being commoner in women than men and in older than in younger people. It involves pain, discomfort or restlessness in the legs, which is at its worst when you are at rest, particularly in the evening, at bedtime and in the early hours. You can't keep your legs still, which makes it difficult to sleep, and they often keep moving periodically even if you do manage to drift off, which as often as not leads to your partner angrily waking you to tell you to keep still. Then the restless sleeplessness starts all over again. Those with the condition are often chronically sleep deprived and drowsy through the day.

Often there is no obvious single cause, but iron deficiency, heavy alcohol and/or caffeine consumption, lack of exercise and some medicines are often implicated. Medicines such as antidepressants, antipsychotic drugs and antihistamines are particular culprits, which is awkward, as insomnia commonly afflicts people with depression and other mental illnesses, meaning that they often need these drugs (sedative antihistamines are often used as low addiction-potential sleeping tablets).

Sleep apnoea

This condition occurs in about 5 per cent of men and 3–4 per cent of women. There is more than one type, but obstructive sleep apnoea is by far the most common. This involves the airway becoming partly blocked during sleep. The affected person's partner will report that he snores, usually quite loudly. The snoring becomes more and more intense and eventually it sounds as if he is choking. Then he stops breathing more or less completely, sometimes for over a minute, ending with him apparently waking gasping for breath. He is often blissfully unaware of the drama which has played out, being in fact still in a light stage of sleep, progressing serenely into a period of normal breathing, only for the whole cycle to start up again once he re-enters the deeper stages of sleep.

People with sleep apnoea (and their partners) tend to be tired all the time, because their normal sleep architecture is severely disrupted. They spend very little time in the restorative deeper stages of sleep, because in deep sleep the relaxation of muscle tone in the pharynx leads to partial airway blockage and consequently a lack of oxygen getting into the body, causing partial or complete waking.

Though women going through the menopause can be vulnerable to sleep apnoea, men are more often affected. Obesity is the principal cause, though some people with sleep apnoea are of normal body weight. Heavy alcohol consumption is again a contributor, as are respiratory disorders such as hay fever, bronchitis and asthma. It sometimes occurs in diabetics and those with other metabolic disorders and can complicate heart disease. It is more common with increasing age and in those on sedative medications such as sleeping tablets and tranquillizers. Diazepam (Valium), being a strong muscle relaxant, may quite often cause or worsen the condition. In some people it seems to happen for no obvious reason at all.

Apart from the chronic tiredness which it causes, sleep apnoea isn't good for you, though the exact degree to which it can contribute to other conditions, such as hypertension (high blood pressure) or impaired glucose metabolism, isn't clear. Recent research suggests it may contribute to an earlier decline in intellectual function than would otherwise occur. Again, whether this means that it can lead to dementia isn't clear as yet. I doubt it.

7

The sleep diary

All right, so we've done the hard part, which is ploughing through most of the factors which may have contributed to your insomnia. But before we move on to what can be done to help you sleep better, we need to get a more objective picture of what the problem really is. This means keeping a sleep diary.

It's a bit counter-intuitive, this, and I always have mixed feelings about getting my patients to record their sleep pattern. Many of them are totally fixated on their sleep and can think about nothing else. Getting them to keep a record of their sleeplessness seems like colluding with this distorted focus on one aspect of their lives to the exclusion of all others. Unfortunately, there really isn't any alternative if we are going to analyse properly the nature and degree of the problem in order to develop an effective treatment plan. It's a temporary measure and won't be needed for long. Once your sleep starts significantly and consistently to improve, so that you are no longer needing to assess the efficacy of the measures taken to improve your sleep, you should put your sleep diary in the bin.

The sleep diary isn't completely accurate, as you fill it in the following morning so you may forget the precise timings, but it is close enough to be useful. It doesn't tell you how much time you spend in each stage of sleep: for example, what proportion of the night is spent in the deeper, most restorative stages. That can only be determined accurately by an electroencephalogram (EEG), which would mean spending a night in a sleep laboratory. In complex cases that is occasionally necessary, but we can usually infer from a well-kept sleep diary roughly how much time is spent in light versus deeper sleep. If long periods are recorded as awake or drowsing, with several episodes of waking in the night, it is likely that much of the total sleep time is in the lighter stages 1 and 2. Likewise, if several dreams are remembered in detail, you have probably woken directly from dreaming on more than one occa-

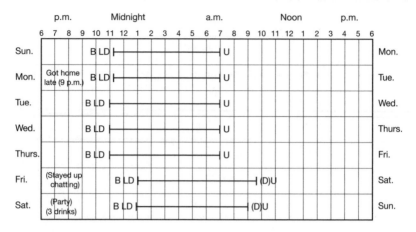

Figure 7.1 Sleep diary for a healthy young adult

B = Gets into bed
L = Lights out
D ( ) = Drowsing. The brackets reflect longer periods of drowsing. Ten minutes or less is represented by a D alone
⊢⊣= Asleep
U = Gets up.

sion in the night, implying that the sleep cycle has probably been at quite a light level overall.

Figure 7.1 shows a typical sleep diary for a healthy young adult.

As I mentioned earlier, drowsing – that is, feeling very drowsy, being still and feeling that it would be difficult to get up or do anything purposeful, being aware of surroundings and sensations but not responding to them – is actually usually stage 1 of sleep.

As you can see, this person goes to bed at some time after 10 p.m. during the working week, reads for 20 minutes or so, then turns out the light. He is drowsing (entering the light stages of sleep) within 10 to 20 minutes and a few minutes later is sleeping soundly, which he does for the rest of the night. He then wakes with the alarm at 6.50 a.m. and gets out of bed shortly after 7 a.m. He stays up late with his partner on Friday and goes out to a party on Saturday night, sleeping in on both Saturday and Sunday mornings.

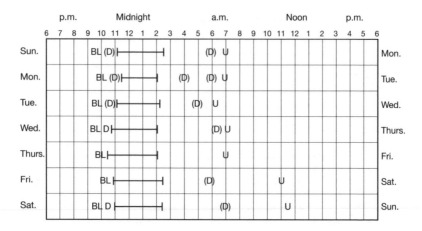

Figure 7.2 Sleep diary for a person with a depressive illness

For an older adult, the total sleep time at night is likely to be reduced, with earlier bedtimes, occasional waking during the night, longer periods of drowsing, earlier rising and for some an occasional brief weekend nap (not recommended if you don't sleep well).

Figure 7.2 shows a sleep diary for someone with a depressive illness.

You will see that the differences in sleep pattern between someone sleeping well and a person with the characteristic sleep loss of major depression are clearly illustrated by these charts. The person with depression is waking in the early morning and is unable fully to get back to sleep. Her total sleep time is reduced to around four hours. Other than about half an hour before her alarm goes off and she has to get up, she isn't really drowsing much. Sometimes she gives up on sleep and gets up before her alarm, but usually she stays in bed for as long as possible as mornings are her worst time and she would like to avoid the world for as long as possible. Her onset of sleep is fairly fast because she is exhausted at the end of the day. She has no energy or enthusiasm to read, so she turns her light off as soon as she goes to bed.

An anxious person, on the contrary, finds difficulty mainly in getting to sleep, though his night may also be interrupted. He does

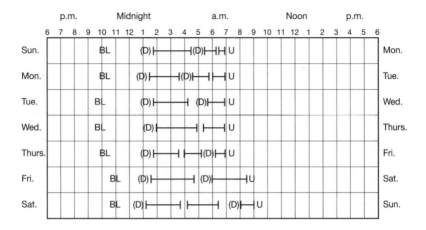

Figure 7.3 Sleep diary for a person with generalized anxiety disorder

not usually have difficulty later in the night and is normally woken by his alarm clock (Figure 7.3).

This chart needs to be kept for every night and a picture of your average sleep pattern built up, including how long you lie awake, your average total hours of sleep and other relevant factors. For example, if you went out for dinner, got home late from work, had several drinks or took a sleeping tablet, these factors need to be written on the record, so that any consistent correlation between them and your sleep pattern can be deduced. Figure 7.4 overleaf shows a typical sleep record for someone who engages in weekend binge drinking. Note the disrupted sleep after an evening's drinking and the reduction in sleep time at night after an afternoon nap.

Once you have at least a week of these records, you should be able to see a pattern to your sleep disturbance, though the longer the period you keep records, the more solid the conclusions you will be able to draw. Look for any correlations between good or bad nights' sleep and situations or habits which you have engaged in. Work out your average total hours of sleep over the period measured, counting drowsing as sleep. If you find drowsing difficult to remember or differentiate from sleep, don't worry. Just record your sleeping and drowsing time all as sleep. You may be unsure when

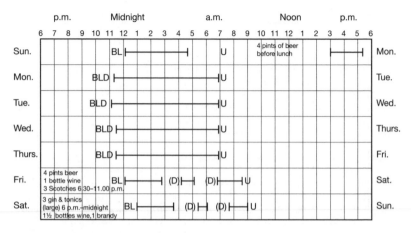

Figure 7.4 Typical sleep diary after heavy weekend alcohol consumption in the evening

you actually fell asleep. If you can't remember it, you were probably sleeping. Sleep laboratory studies show that most people significantly underestimate their time asleep.

Once this has been done and you have worked out which of the causes of insomnia I have listed apply to you, we will be in a position to decide on a plan to improve your sleep.

As an aside, you may find that your sleep pattern changes when you start measuring it. There are two reasons for this. First, it is one of the basic tenets of science that as soon as you measure something, you change it. This applies to sleep as much as anything else. Second, measuring your sleep disturbance may allow you to stop fighting it, essentially allowing you to accept it. Acceptance of insomnia takes away some of its power, making you less fearful of it and so less over-aroused.

8

How can I sleep better?
I: Managing stress

By this point, having analysed the nature of your sleep problem and the causes behind it, the remedies may be obvious. Deal with the causes and the problem resolves itself. The biggest of these contributors is stress, so before I go on to more specific measures to improve sleep, I need to touch on some of what you need to change in order to be less stressed.

Look back at Chapter 5 and have a think about what causes your stress. I separated out external from internal causes of stress. This doesn't mean that we only have influence over what is internal, or caused by us. There are choices in everything, each choice having its own natural consequences.

It is true that the world is more stressful than it used to be and that change is constant. That's just the way the world is nowadays. But we don't have to buy into it. A degree of selective cynicism is helpful here. Don't be cynical about the things which really matter in your job, your family or your friendships, but do be about the nonsense, the politicians, the silly diktats of the latest restructured management team and today's screaming tabloid headline. As a journalist once told me: 'All we care about is a good story. If it happens to be true, all the better.'

Do what you have to in order to stay under the radar and concentrate on what really matters in your life. If your place of work makes you sick, think about what your choices are. Do you *really* have to stay? Are you sure? Think long and hard before you answer that one. If you are taking all of the circumstances and privileges of your salary and your job as a given, you have constructed a prison cell for yourself. There is a doorway out of your cell, with no lock on the door, and the doorway is marked 'Guilt'. Making choices, whether to leave your well-paid but hated job or to change any other given in order to seek a better, freer and simpler life, is the biggest single change which you can make in seeking less stress, more happiness and better sleep.

Get comfortable with mistakes and failure. I don't mean seek them out, but recognize and accept that if you are extending and challenging yourself you are going to slip up sometimes. Accept this, do your best, learn from your mistakes and *refuse to beat yourself up*. This is true accountability and it works. When I was at school, they used to hit us with a stick when we got things wrong. We don't do that any more, partly because it is morally wrong but also partly because it doesn't work. It's inefficient. A good teacher points out kindly to his pupil that he has made a mistake and shows him how to correct it, demonstrating the satisfying result of employing the correct method, thus infusing the pupil with enthusiasm and motivation. The same is true for adults. Punishment doesn't work, leading only to powerlessness and apathy; and insulting yourself for your mistakes and shortcomings is a punishment. Avoid double standards here. Ensure that you only ever say to yourself what you would say to an honoured and cherished friend. Insults aren't all right even if they are only directed by you towards yourself.

Almost as toxic as the beatings you give yourself are the people who call themselves friends but who really just use and abuse you. I define a friend as someone who is friendly. If they aren't friendly, focusing on themselves to the exclusion of you and your feelings, they aren't friends. A relatively empty address book may be lonely for a while, but if you keep the users and abusers away and look out for the givers, they will eventually arrive.

Empowering yourself is the opposite of beating yourself up. It means making active choices based on what *you* want, not what others say you should want, allowing yourself to make mistakes because you don't have hindsight in advance, asking yourself 'What is it all for?' and actively looking for a balance in your life which allows space for a creative search for what you find beautiful.

Accept who you are. Don't try to be the person you feel you should be or, even worse, the person your critical parent wanted you to be, unless you really want to achieve this and it is realistically achievable. If you didn't ever get the approval of your father, *it never was you, it was him*. A parent is supposed to give his child unconditional love and affirmation. If you didn't get that, it was because of his failings, not yours. He was emotionally disabled. Inside you is a sad and frightened child who needs love, respect and reassurance. There's only one person who is in a position to deliver the child's needs and it's you. Strive to be at ease with the person you are.

Even if you are a parent, wanting to put your children first, remember that it's in their interests to see you care for yourself as well as them. You are modelling a behaviour which, hopefully, they will copy later in life, which says, 'You matter enormously to me, but I matter too.' Remember, a 'good enough' parent is better than a perfect one.

Stress doesn't create the symptoms linked with it, including insomnia: you do. Weak, cynical, lazy, manipulative or selfish people don't tend to suffer from stress. People around them do but they don't, because they always ensure that life suits them. I'm not suggesting that you become like that, but we can learn something from everyone, including the bad guy. It's about balance. If you are determined that you are going to keep everybody happy all the time you are going to suffer from stress, because it's impossible. Their unhappiness belongs to them, not to you. Accepting your limitations and letting people sometimes be disappointed with you without trying to fix it are crucial steps on the path to overcoming stress.

In the same way, stress is caused by trying too hard to control life. I've already discussed in Chapter 5 the importance of letting life be. The Serenity Prayer of that excellent body, Alcoholics Anonymous, gets it right: 'God, give me the serenity to accept what I can't change, the strength to change what I can and the wisdom to know the difference between the two.' Putting it another way is this example, taken from my earlier book *Stress-Related Illness*. A passenger on a coach trip through beautiful countryside decides that he wants to control the route taken. He leaps out of his chair, goes to the front of the coach, pushes aside the driver and takes the wheel. Oh please, go and sit down! You aren't going to experience any of the lovely scenery while you're driving. If you return to your seat, you may not be in control of the route but you'll experience so many interesting sights along the way. Life is so much more fun and interesting if you go along for the ride. I'll return to this theme under the heading of 'Mindfulness' in the next chapter (page 51).

Choose your battles carefully. Avoid right-fighting when you can. Accept that feelings are neither right nor wrong. You and your partner are both entitled to your feelings and to express them. Only defend yourself when you have to. There's nothing as disarming as having one's feelings acknowledged, and doing so isn't an admission of wrongdoing. Work on negotiating your needs, respectfully, stating your wishes clearly and assertively and accepting that if they conflict with those of your partner, a compromise may need to be sought.

Try to minimize your value judgements (see Chapter 5), particularly about yourself, and don't look for fairness but search instead for opportunities. I've never met a happy person who looks for fairness, as the world isn't constructed that way. If you can accept this, you'll find that from time to time life throws you a bouquet which you haven't earned. It cuts both ways.

Use alcohol only for the purpose for which it is best designed, that is as occasional social recreation. It's a lousy tranquillizer and a worse sleeping aid.

Remember that exercise is an effective stress-reliever so long as it is used moderately. Exercise regularly, but not excessively or too late in the evening, as you need a few hours of quiet restfulness before bed to allow your arousal level to fall and to enable a transition into sleep. What you are after is exercise sufficient to make you slightly out of breath (aerobic), but not in pain or totally exhausted.

Try to simplify your life, giving priority to what really matters. There is a parable about a teacher who fills a bell jar to the top with rocks.

'Is it full?' he asks his class.

'Yes,' replies a student, whereupon the teacher pours a load of pebbles around the rocks.

'It wasn't full, but is it now?' he asks.

'Yes, now it is full,' says another student. The teacher pours sand around the rocks and pebbles.

'Now it really is full,' asserts a third student. The teacher pours a can of beer into the jar, perfectly filling it to the rim.

'The jar is your life,' explains the teacher. 'The sand is those routines and chores you spend so much of your life on, like bills, washing, preparing meals and such like. The pebbles are the important stuff, like family, friends and work. The rocks are those parts of life which really give it meaning, which give you fun and joy, maybe music, sport, art or whatever.'

He fills a second jar with sand. There is no space for any rocks or pebbles.

'Put the rocks in first. That is the key to a happy life.'

'But what was the meaning of the can of beer?' asks a student.

'Ah,' replies the sage. 'That just shows that, however full your life may be, there's always room for a beer.'

Yes, I know, I warned against using alcohol regularly – but occasionally popping out to the pub for a pint with a friend does no harm. It's all part of a moderate, balanced life.

There's more detail on these topics in my book *Stress-Related Illness*, if you need it. If you think you may need a therapist or counsellor to help you with some of this stuff, go and speak to your GP, who may be able to access one through the NHS. For now, what I want to emphasize is that managing your stress may be the most important factor in improving your sleep. In Chapter 9, I will enlarge on three of the most important techniques in managing stress and improving stress-related insomnia: challenging unhelpful thoughts and beliefs, mindfulness and relaxation training.

9

How can I sleep better?
II: Managing your mind

Because night-time is when nothing else crowds in on your brain, as it does through the day, this is when your mind tends to go into overdrive if you let it, or if you don't know how to keep it quiet. Getting really good at managing your mind is central to improving your sleep. This means getting expert at a relaxation exercise, at how to be mindful and at how to challenge the unhelpful and unrealistic thinking patterns which keep you awake.

Relaxation

Relaxation exercises can be immensely powerful if persevered with, allowing you to bring your level of arousal down to a level which allows you to drift off to sleep. There are many variations on this theme and the thing is to find the one which works best for you. There are several relaxation exercises commercially available as audio files, on CD or other spoken-word media. Some people get benefit from yoga techniques learnt in a group setting. Others find that following a written set of instructions helps them better, by allowing them to do the exercise at their own pace with their own mental imagery. What follows is just one example of such a technique, but one which many of my patients have found helpful, whether they are affected by insomnia or any other stress-related symptom.

Whichever way you choose, the essential point is that it needs a lot of practice. Though a few people pick it up very quickly, for the majority, relaxation exercises are a total waste of time *to begin with*. They don't work straight away, leading many to become disillusioned and give up on them. Some people even feel worse at the beginning, because doing anything and having it fail tends to make you feel tense.

Persevere, because when you really master the technique you will find that it changes your life. You're doing it not to get benefit from it yet, but as an investment in your future. In the absence of any other strategy, expertise in relaxation may be all you need to get your sleep pattern back. The people who get benefit from relaxation exercises are those who put them top of their list of priorities and practise for at least half an hour every day, come hell or high water. If you hear that a meteor is going to vaporize your town in 24 hours, by all means take flight for the hills, but not until you've done your relaxation practice.

Looking back, I did relaxation exercises every day for about three years, not because I was unusually anxious but because I thought then, as now, that everybody can benefit from them. It took me about a month of daily practice for the exercise to be of any use at all. It took me at least three months to get to the stage of being able to use it when I was under strain, such as before an exam, because the most difficult time to do a relaxation exercise is when you most need it, at times of high stress. In about two to three years I got to the stage of no longer needing the exercise because I could switch on a relaxed state like a light when necessary. I'm a bit slow, as I'm told that the average time to get that good is about nine months, but never mind, I got there in the end and it changed my life. I can tell you first hand that it's worth all the time and effort.

A relaxation exercise

Spend 20–30 minutes on this exercise.

1 Find a suitable place to relax. A bed or easy chair is ideal but anywhere will do, preferably quiet and private. Once you are good enough at the exercise to find it useful, do it when you go to bed.
2 Try to clear your mind of thoughts as far as you can.
3 Take three very slow, very deep breaths (10–15 seconds to breathe in and out once).
4 Imagine a neutral figure. An example may be the number 1. Don't choose any object or figure with emotional significance, such as a ring or a person, for example. Let it fill your mind. See it in your mind's eye, give it a colour, try to see it in 3D

and repeat it to yourself under your breath, many times over. Continue until it fills your mind.

5 Slowly change to imagine yourself in a quiet, peaceful and pleasant place or situation. This may be a favourite place or situation, or a pleasant scene from your past. Be there and notice all the feelings, in each sense. See it, feel it, hear it, smell it and taste it. Spend some time there.

6 Slowly change to be aware of your body. Notice any tension in your body. Take each group of muscles in turn and tense, then relax them two or three times each. Include fingers, hands, arms, shoulders, neck, face, chest, tummy, buttocks, thighs, legs, feet and toes. Be aware of the feeling of relaxation in contrast to how the tense muscles felt. When complete, spend some time in this relaxed state. If you aren't relaxed, don't worry; you're just practising for now.

7 Slowly get up and go about your business if you're doing the exercise during the day. If it's bedtime, just lie in bed until you drop off to sleep (this is when you're good at it; to begin with, remember, it may not work).

At step 5, I want to emphasize that this isn't simply visualization. It is a multi-sensory experience. Let me demonstrate. You are imagining yourself on a beautiful Caribbean beach. Lovely. But that isn't

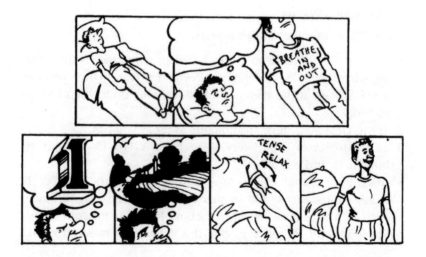

enough. Which direction is the wind coming from? Is it constant or puffy? What does it feel like when the sun goes behind a cloud? Does it get cooler? What does hot sun on sand smell of and what is the smell of your suntan lotion? Is the sand soft or hard? How do the waves sound? What does your drink taste of? How far back does the grass start? Are the palm trees small stumpy palms or tall coconut palms? If they are coconut palms, are the coconuts brown or green?

You need to be there in every sense. This takes quite a lot of practice.

Don't hurry this procedure, and remember to practise. It will work.

Mindfulness

Mindfulness, or mindfulness-based cognitive behavioural therapy (MBCBT), is a very powerful technique. Many would say that it's more than that, being a whole way of life. It's a way of being which has been lifted from Buddhist philosophy and taken on by the cognitive therapy movement. I'm only going to touch on it here as, if the concept interests you, I would suggest that you invest in one of the excellent texts on the subject written by an expert. I would recommend *Wherever You Go, There You Are: Mindfulness Meditation for Everyday Life* by Jon Kabat-Zinn (London: Piatkus, 2004), *Mindfulness: A Practical Guide to Finding Peace in a Frantic World* by Mark Williams and Danny Penman (London: Piatkus, 2011), or any one of the myriad books on mindfulness for sleep that you will find online or at a good bookseller.

In principle, mindfulness is beautifully simple, though in practice it can be difficult to carry out. Again, it's all about practice. There are only two main principles. The first is *stay present*. Don't spend time ruminating about the past, except when you are trying to learn positive lessons from it. There is a time for reflection and learning from experience, but not repetitively and not at night. Once a period of reflection has led to appropriate conclusions, you need to come straight back into the present. Don't then revisit the past event unless something new has happened or changed, requiring further re-evaluation. Equally, don't ruminate about the future unless you are doing real planning. When the plan is made, come straight back into the present. The stuff you're worrying about won't happen anyway, though something else will, and there will be time to deal with that, whatever it is, when it happens. Your miserable meandering through your past and your future is a set of myths created by your distorted take on things. The only reality available to you is *now*, so experience it. This means being really conscious of your situation and environment, of everything which you perceive and feel. What colour are the flowers you have just passed? What does the birdsong sound like? What colour are the bricks of the house in front of you? The list of sensations available to you is long, if you are really conscious and notice them.

The second principle of mindfulness is *stop fighting*: that is, accept what is and can't be changed. In order to experience life we have to stop fighting it. So stop fighting the past, the future, unfairness, people, institutions, symptoms and, most of all, your insomnia.

The mindful solution to insomnia is to experience your wakefulness; not to fight it, not to worry what the consequences of it might be, but to accept and experience being awake, now. This is the opposite of *trying to sleep*. It is giving in to it, or appearing to. Several Eastern martial arts include the concept of defeating your opponent by appearing to submit to him. If you are unfortunate enough to be confronted by a man running towards you with a knife, the best thing you can do is to position yourself in front of a wall. As your assailant gets almost to touching distance, you step deftly to one side, allowing him to crash headlong into the wall. Through your quiet refusal to engage in combat, your opponent has defeated himself. Your victory against insomnia will come, not through struggle, but through the lack of it.

I know this sounds easier said than done and maybe it is, but mindfully accepting and experiencing your insomnia is much better for your well-being than fighting with it and, paradoxically, is much more likely to lead to sleep. Mindfulness is calmness, calmness is low arousal and low arousal leads in due course to sleep. Your sleeplessness isn't present because you're neglecting to *do* something, it's because what you are doing and thinking is getting in sleep's way.

Like relaxation techniques, mindfulness takes practice. Do get one of the books I've mentioned, go to some mindfulness classes, get a mindfulness audio-file or whatever, but stick at it.

Cognitive behavioural therapy (CBT) for insomnia

Much of what I have already discussed in this chapter and will discuss in Chapter 10 is incorporated in what many sleep clinics call cognitive therapy, but in this section I want to focus on dealing with unhelpful thinking patterns and associated behaviours.

There are two types of unhelpful thoughts which interfere with sleep. These are (1) intrusive thoughts about your waking life and (2) specific erroneous thoughts about sleep and insomnia.

Examples of (1) are: 'What am I going to say at tomorrow's important meeting?', 'I'm sure I'll forget to buy the cat food tomorrow; how can I be sure to remember?' or 'That guy at work was really rude to me today. Tomorrow I'm going to give him a real mouthful.'

These types of thoughts are fairly easily dealt with, through the repository of thoughts and the principle of nocturnal forgiveness.

The repository of thoughts

The repository of thoughts is a notepad and pen on your bedside table. Make it a fairly big notepad and ensure that the pen and paper are easy to put your hands on in the dark, well away from your glass of water, because you're going to be writing with the light off. At the top of the sheet of paper is a time period in the morning (say 6.30–7.00 a.m.) when you will consider the thoughts you have written down. Each time one of these thoughts pops into your head, write it on the pad. The next morning, at the appointed time, go through your list of thoughts and consider them. This will allow the pop-up mechanism in your brain (see Chapter 3) to delete this thought for the night. When you look at your list of thoughts in the morning the chances are that they will look fairly silly and blown out of proportion, because things always seem worse in the night than in the cool light of day, but consider them you must, otherwise the next night, when you write your thoughts down, your brain won't believe that you'll really deal with them the next day, so it will keep popping them back into your head. I've had to

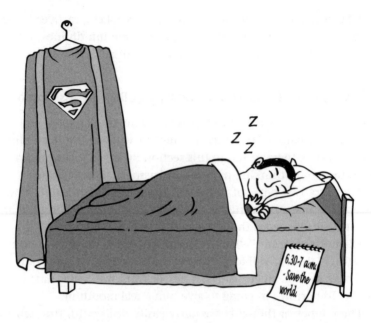

use a repository of thoughts myself while writing this book, because ideas of what to add to the text tend to pop into my head when I wake up at night. It works well for me, allowing me to go back to sleep secure in the knowledge that my nocturnal brainwave won't be forgotten by the morning.

Nocturnal forgiveness

Nocturnal forgiveness may sound rather like a pious idea, impractical in the ferociously competitive modern world, but it's really important and, like everything else, is a matter of practice. Whether in the morning you plan the sadistic murder of the object of your anger is no business of mine, but at night-time everyone is forgiven everything. Use the repository of thoughts to store your resentment for the morning if you need to, but *never* allow yourself angry thoughts at night-time. If they come into your mind, actively replace them with forgiveness. This may be easier for people with a religious faith, but it's possible for anyone, given time and perseverance. I know this from experience, not being one of the most forgiving of people myself, but being fairly diligent in practising new skills.

Even more important than forgiving others is forgiving yourself. Do you tend to beat yourself up for things you feel you've got wrong? If so, this is a case of double standards, as you wouldn't treat anybody else to this level of abusive criticism. There is a frightened and vulnerable child inside you who needs kindness and reassurance, not criticism and abuse, particularly at bedtime. The person best placed to deliver this kindness is you. You need to practise challenging your unfair self-criticism, probably decanting your thoughts into the next day using your repository of thoughts. At bedtime only kindness is allowed.

Dealing with erroneous thoughts about sleep and insomnia

Unhelpful thoughts of type (2) can be a bit more complicated to deal with. Common thoughts of this type are:

- I've got to sleep well tonight, or I won't be able to perform tomorrow.
- I have to sleep eight hours each night.
- If I sleep poorly I'll get ill.
- I'm in despair: I'll never sleep well again.
- If I don't sleep well, I'll be tired all day and won't cope.
- I've already been awake for two hours when I should have been asleep; I've got to get to sleep now.
- My insomnia is a big worry, it'll ruin my life.
- I'll need to take a long nap tomorrow to make up for the sleep I've lost.
- I'd better take it easy tomorrow, as my lost sleep means I'll need to conserve my energy and strength.
- I'd better keep checking the alarm clock to see how much sleep I've lost.
- I feel dreadful – look at what insomnia does to you.
- I can't sleep without medication.
- My sleeplessness is caused by a chemical imbalance so there's nothing I can do about it.

These are just some of the common sleep-wrecking thoughts. They are all unrealistic, but you may have to check that out for yourself. Have a really good think about it. What are the thoughts which cause you worry about your sleep pattern? List them. Now think of some alternatives to your worrying assumptions. Write these down too. Do they make more sense than your worries? Give the alternative thoughts a percentage probability rating. Remember all that you read earlier in this book about sleep, how it works and the relative importance of not sleeping versus worry in causing malaise and other symptoms. In order to find out which alternative thought is correct, you may need to check it out, by way of a behavioural experiment. There's no need to do this if a moment's realistic reflection shows you that the alternative thought is much more likely than your worrying assumption, but if you really believe your negative thoughts then you need to go through this process in order to enable you to think realistically about your sleep.

For example: 'If I don't sleep well, I'll be tired all day and won't cope.' All right, let's see. Keep a record tomorrow of all the time that you feel tired and all the time you don't. If, when something comes up that interests you, you forget your tiredness, your argument has been disproven. 'I rest my case, your honour,' says I. 'Case dismissed,' rules the judge. Don't bother coming up with that argument again, it isn't true. Remember to tell yourself that the next time it comes into your head.

It is useful to write down the results of your behavioural experiments and to re-read them from time to time (Table 9.1).

It may also be worth checking your negative thoughts about sleep with your sleep diary. Are your assumptions about your sleep based on fact, or are your worries out of kilter with your real sleep pattern?

I've already really dealt with the other common misconceptions listed in the bullet points above, but for what it's worth I'll briefly list my counter-arguments here, in the same bullet order as I listed the common thought distortions:

- There is little evidence that one night's poor sleep has more than a minor effect on performance the next day, if you don't worry about it.
- Everyone is different in terms of how much sleep they need and you need less as you get older. Nobody needs eight hours every single night.
- While long-term insomnia can have harmful effects on health,

Table 9.1 A sleep thought record

Thought (A)	Alternative (B)	Per cent probability (A)	Per cent probability (B)	Result of behavioural experiment	Revised probability (A)	Revised probability (B)
I can't sleep without medication.	When I used no sleeping pills for ten days my sleep improved after a few nights, so I can sleep without them.	0	100	–	–	–
If I don't sleep well, I'll be tired all day and won't cope.	I'll be able to do what I need to do even if I'm tired, and I'll only be tired some of the time.	80	20	My sleep diary shows I slept only three hours, but my boss said my presentation was good. I only felt tired for two hours after lunch. I can cope after a bad night's sleep.	10	90

there is no evidence of such harm for short-term sleep problems lasting days or weeks.

- Saying you'll never sleep again is the opposite of mindfulness. Stay in the present and stop creating unpleasant fantasies. *Life-long insomnia is very rare; you're more likely to win the Lottery.*

- After a night's poor sleep, there may be periods of drowsiness, but most people are able to pull things together for limited periods to function pretty well the next day, and when something grabs your attention you tend to forget your tiredness.

- You'll sleep when you sleep. You can't sleep by demanding it. Just concentrate on resting.

- Insomnia won't ruin your life. The only thing which could is your worry. Deal with your worrying and things will get better.

- Don't nap the day after a bad night. If you do, you're setting up the next bad night. Get through the day and leave sleeping to night-time.

- Exercise, so long as it's not taken too near bedtime, promotes sleep. Don't laze around all day after a bad night's sleep: try to be active and tire yourself out.

- Don't keep checking the alarm clock. It keeps you awake. You'll sleep when you sleep. Your hyper-vigilance and checking is part of the problem. Having said this, if you've been awake a long time, you may need to check the clock once if you are practising stimulus control (see Chapter 10).

- If you're feeling dreadful it's because you're worn out from worrying. It isn't the lack of sleep but worrying about your lack of sleep which is grinding you down.

- The best available evidence suggests that while medication may help sleep in the short term, it has no lasting benefit, while the sort of techniques which I'm describing here have been shown to bring enduring benefit to many. What's more, there is no evidence that, in the long term, psychological treatments plus medication work any better than psychological treatments alone (see Chapter 11).

- There's plenty you can do about insomnia. This argument is like saying that because diabetes is chemical, a diabetic can't do any-thing to help herself be healthy. Of course she can. Most of the measures I'm listing in this book have a strong body of evidence behind them and I've seen all of them work well.

You may have other unhelpful thinking patterns interfering with your sleep. Challenge them in the way I've suggested. Hopefully you'll agree that most of the counter-arguments which I've listed here are fairly obvious when you think about it. I suspect that your distorted beliefs about sleep will be just as easy to challenge if you give them some critical thought. If not, talk to your GP about them. She will probably be able to reassure you.

10

How can I sleep better? III: Specific non-pharmacological treatments

In addition to getting really good at managing stress and 'running less hot', there are a number of specific measures you can take to improve your sleep without using medications. These are all based on sound evidence and, unlike drugs, if they work for you their benefit is enduring.

Sleep hygiene

No, I don't mean washing before bedtime, though, as it happens, a lot of people find that having a hot bath before bed helps them to get to sleep. It's the relaxation you get from lying in the bath which does the trick, though it's also possible that the dilation of superficial blood vessels caused by the heat (white people are pink when they get out of the bath), pulling blood away from the brain, may contribute to the drowsiness. It's worth trying, though what 'sleep hygiene' really refers to is doing things which promote sleep at the right time and avoiding doing things which interfere with a normal sleep cycle.

The other measure which probably works by reducing cerebral blood supply is taking a hot milky drink at bedtime. Full fat or semi-skimmed milk probably works better than skimmed milk (so long as you don't have a medical reason to have a low-fat diet), and make sure that there is nothing stimulating in the drink, such as coffee, tea, cocoa or hot chocolate. It is probably that the heat and the fat content of the drink pulls blood into the stomach and gut, thus slightly reducing cerebral blood flow. In fact the brain is protected against lack of blood supply; if you lose blood, the body ensures that the brain is the last organ to go without a blood supply. However, even a slight reduction of blood flow to the brain makes you drowsy, so the hot milky drink is remarkably effective for some.

Caffeine, as mentioned earlier, hangs around in the body for a long time, so you need to limit your consumption of tea and coffee. If you have a sleep problem, I think you should limit yourself to two cups of coffee or three of tea per day and avoid any caffeine-containing drink after 1 p.m. This includes colas and most energy drinks. Also beware of over-the-counter analgesics, as many contain caffeine. Make your afternoon beverage decaffeinated if you need one. I know that this is counter-intuitive; because of your poor sleep, you rely on tea and coffee to keep you going through the day, but you're storing up more insomnia by relying on this drug. Managing your caffeine consumption is important. Other stimulants, such as amphetamines (speed), cocaine, ecstasy or any of the 'legal highs' are an absolute no-no. There is evidence that smoking near bedtime interferes with sleep, so if you do smoke, try to have a gap between your last cigarette and bedtime if possible. If you are on any prescribed medications which you find stimulant or which interfere with sleep in any other way, ask your doctor if you can take them earlier in the day. For example, some antidepressants can cause vivid dreams which can wake you up.

Even more important is managing your intake of alcohol. As I explained earlier in the book (page 19), alcohol may seem to help your sleep but in fact it wrecks it. It is a lousy sleeping draught; don't use it for this purpose. It is true that when you cut back or stop drinking your sleep may temporarily get worse, but in the long term, within a few weeks, it will improve. If you are a very heavy drinker (over a bottle of wine, four pints of ordinary strength beer or a quarter of a bottle of spirits a day), you may need medical help with stopping drinking and doing so abruptly could be hazardous, so see your GP first. For the rest of us, it's using alcohol only for occasional social recreation, in very moderate amounts. Any more than one standard drink may interfere with the architecture of your sleep. Unless there's a good reason not to, it's probably better in fact to avoid the stuff until you are satisfied that your sleep problem is fixed. In any case, any sleeping medication will interact with alcohol, so they shouldn't be taken together.

It's fine to have a glass of water by your bed, but don't drink large amounts of water before bedtime, as it will wake you up once or more in the night to go to the loo. As you get older this will probably happen anyway. Try to do what you have to do with as little fuss as possible. If you can safely get to the toilet with the light off, do so. Otherwise close your eyes once you're sitting on the throne. Asssuming you wash in the morning, I would even suggest that hand-washing can be fairly cursory following nocturnal urination, if the idea doesn't horrify you.

Your bedroom environment is important. Having the heat on and the window open may seem wasteful, but it sometimes makes sense. There is evidence that a significantly raised carbon dioxide concentration in air can interfere with sleep. This can occur in a stuffy bedroom. Being either too hot or too cold can be equally destructive. Unless it's a really cold winter, it's probably fine to have the heating turn off shortly after you're snuggled up under your cosy duvet or blankets, but if you regularly need to get up in the night you may need to programme the heating to stay on.

Your bedroom also needs to be dark and quiet. The former should be doable, by getting good thick curtains, blinds or shutters or, if that isn't possible, by using an eye mask. The latter may be harder if there is often noise outside where you sleep, or if your partner snores. I'm sorry if this seems unromantic, but it may be worth using another quieter room to sleep in for a while, until you're sleeping better, if you have this luxury. Otherwise it's earplugs. The foam ones don't work; probably best to use the more expensive silicone or wax ones, though find what works for you. Also, avoid having your clock facing you directly. If it has a bright LCD display or a luminous face, this can give off quite a lot of light and it encourages you to check the time regularly. You need to reduce your monitoring of your sleeplessness, so don't make it easy to keep checking the time. You may need to do so occasionally (see 'Stimulus control' on page 65), but having at least to turn the clock to see it is a good idea.

Don't have a TV in the bedroom and don't watch thrillers, sports or anything else which gets you going within two hours of going to bed. In particular, don't deal with problems near bedtime. Yes, I know that's very hard if you have kids, but it is really important.

Try to find a way of putting problem-solving off to another time if it is at all possible.

If you're having a row near bedtime, see if you can agree to call a time out and revisit the issue tomorrow. That's a whole new area which may need another book: how to deal with rows. We have to look at it now, though, as rows tend to happen in the evening, because that's when the children are in bed and there's time to talk, and it's when we drink. If you have a sparky relationship and you don't sleep well, you need to work out a different time to discuss difficult or contentious issues. The bottom line is this: you aren't going to sleep soon after a row. If you have them quite often and they happen in the evening, there's your problem. Have a chat with your partner and work out a strategy, before 6 p.m., if this is an issue for you.

Read something in bed which isn't too exciting. *National Geographic* magazine or some such pleasantly interesting publication will do, but anything relating to your work or any passionately held interest or hobby won't. I've been reading, on and off, a book by Marcel Proust called *Remembrance of Things Past* for about twenty years now. It's in several volumes amounting to over a thousand pages, of which I've read a few hundred of the first one. Nothing has happened yet, but it's a beautiful book, very well written, and I find it helps me to sleep when I need it to.

Think about the things, personal to you, which make you calm. These are the things which make you go 'Aahh', which bring a smile to your lips, unhunch your shoulders and take your frown away. This really is different for everyone. For me it's hitting a perfect golf shot, the taste of that perfect glass of wine, or the day I married my wife on the beach at Cape Cod with Hurricane Isobel in attendance. It doesn't sound calming, but it is to me. For you it may be your favourite car, sex, shoes, money, flowers, anything. It's what gives you peace. These thoughts may be part of a relaxation exercise or used on their own. If worries get in the way, use your repository of thoughts (see Chapter 9). If you find gentle sounds, such as waves breaking or rain falling, are calming, there are a number of devices available which produce these sounds as a background for sleep. Others find having the radio on softly in the background helps; if it works for you and you sleep alone, do it.

Try to make your bedroom a simple, uncluttered place, used for only two purposes: sleep and, if relevant, sex. Not eating, texting or emailing, and absolutely not work. If you can afford it, get a really good, comfortable mattress, and if you sleep with a partner, make sure the bed is big enough. As I mentioned earlier in the book, sex may either wake you up or make you sleepy. I don't wish to be prurient here, but let's just say that you should plan your activities accordingly.

Keep regular habits. Your circadian rhythm depends on them. This means, where possible, regular mealtimes. Don't go to bed over-full and avoid spicy foods for supper, especially if you tend to indigestion or heartburn. It also means regular exercise at the same time each day (not too near bedtime), avoiding using the phone or attending to any tasks requiring brain power late at night and allowing a period of non-productive rest before going to bed at roughly the same time each evening. This sounds terribly boring, but once you've been sleeping well for a while you can take a few more liberties with your body clock. The only situation in which it is worth breaking this constant routine is if you're really wound up just before bedtime, for example by a phone call or something you've read. In this situation, do some relaxation, meditation, reading or listening to calming music until you've settled down.

If you have a dimmer switch in your sitting room, turn the dimmer down later in the evening. If not, get some lower wattage bulbs. Bright light in the late evening is worth avoiding because it switches on the SCN (see Chapter 2).

Be realistic about what you expect from your sleeping pattern. I dealt with this in Chapter 2, so revisit it if you need to. Don't expect to sleep like you did thirty years ago or like someone else who has always slept like a log. Accepting the limits of your sleeping pattern will help to make it as good as it can be, though maybe not as good as you'd wish it was.

Above all, however strong the temptation, *don't take daytime naps*. If you do, your sleep at night won't improve. Don't even sleep in at the weekend when you've had a bad night. It's really important that you re-establish a regular sleep pattern, including consistent times of going to bed and getting up in the morning. Sleeping at any unusual times will prevent this.

Stimulus control

This strategy is all about persuading your brain that the bedroom is where you sleep. It's based on the conditioning model: that is, repetitively linking two stimuli such that eventually the one automatically leads to the other. If you repeatedly lie awake in bed for long periods, going to bed will lead to wakefulness, not sleep. Conversely, if you only stay in the bedroom when you are sleeping, your brain will link bed with sleepiness and turn on the sleep response when you go there.

Different sleep experts advise different periods, but the point is that after you have been lying in bed awake for a certain length of time, you get up and go to another room. I would suggest 30 minutes as a reasonable length of time to give it before you get up. Remember that drowsing (being sleepy, not active, but vaguely aware of your surroundings) is often actually light sleep, so don't take this too literally. If you're beginning to drift off, you don't have to get up on the dot of half an hour. In any case, you may feel that this advice conflicts with what I said earlier about not checking your bedside clock regularly. You just need to find a reasonable balance. If you've been in bed fully awake for quite a while, which feels like half an hour or so, check the clock, and if you were right, get up and go to another room. Don't check the clock every two minutes to ensure you get up exactly on the half hour though.

Make sure the room you go to has dim lighting and is quiet, warm and comfortable. The dim lighting, with no LCD or TV screen on, is important, as we need to switch off your SCN, your 'on-button', which responds to light. By all means read something of the type I described earlier in this chapter, or leaf through a magazine. Alternatively just sit and rest or practise a relaxation or mindfulness exercise, but try not to ruminate about problems, do anything useful or lie down. If necessary, take your repository of thoughts with you and write down any ruminations which keep popping back into your head.

When you start to feel sleepy again, go back to bed. Then the same rule applies. You may have to go through more than one cycle of going to bed, getting up, then going back to bed again.

However, over days or weeks, this strategy usually leads to the bedroom becoming a place where you feel sleepy and sleep usually improves.

Sleep restriction

Like several of the measures in this book, this seems counter-intuitive. If you can't sleep you don't want to reduce your time in bed, do you? Well, yes, actually you probably do. We're not going to increase your hours asleep instantly, but if we can get you to feel sleepy at bedtime, we'll succeed in the end. We need to increase your sleep load (see Chapter 2). We do this by reducing your time resting in bed. It also helps with stimulus control: that is, getting the brain to link the bedroom with sleep. Sleep restriction is a controversial strategy, but it can be very effective.

Here's where your sleep diary becomes particularly important. Look back over the last week of your diary and work out your average sleep time (average time asleep: ATA). For seven days, that is your total hours of sleep plus drowsing over this period, divided by seven. Take this figure and add 20 per cent. This is the length of time you should be spending in bed (time in bed: TIB). Stay with me on this, it isn't as technical and mathematical as it sounds. If your ATA is five hours, your TIB should be five hours plus 20 per cent, that is five hours plus one-fifth of five hours (one hour), which equals six hours.

You don't have to be exact on this; take it to the nearest half an hour.

Taking the example above, say you tend to go to bed at 10 p.m. and get up at 7 a.m., you're spending nine hours in bed, but only sleeping for five of them. You're going to have to lop three hours off that, maybe going to bed at 11 p.m. and setting the alarm for 5 a.m. I know this sounds scary and you will probably feel more tired for a while but, as they say, you can't make an omelette without breaking eggs.

After a week of this, look at your sleep diary again. If it's working and your ATA is increasing, you can increase your TIB accordingly, using the same TIB equals ATA plus 20 per cent algorithm. If you slept the full six hours, or near to it, your TIB next week will be six hours plus 20 per cent, or about seven hours. Hooray, an extra hour in bed!

If it isn't working and your ATA isn't increasing, you need to restrict your sleep further, to ATA plus 10 per cent. That means if your ATA is five hours, your TIB now needs to be reduced to five hours plus 10 per cent (one-tenth), which equals five and a half hours. If you're going to bed at 11 p.m., that means the alarm is now set for 4.30 a.m.

This pattern gets reset once a week. If there's no increase in ATA by the end of the second week, TIB goes down to ATA plus 5 per cent, where it stays until there is progress. Before long, you should find that it's difficult to stay awake until your appointed bedtime. If so, give yourself a little bit of latitude with the rule, but not too much. If you get excited and go back straight away, as soon as you see some improvement, to your old bedtime and morning alarm time, you'll probably go back to not sleeping. If in doubt, it's better to stick to the rule, wait to the end of the week and then, if the ATA has risen at all, even slightly, the next week's TIB goes back up from ATA plus 5 per cent to ATA plus 10 per cent. If the next week it improves again, the TIB is back up to ATA plus 20 per cent, where it stays for as long as you are keeping your sleep diary – that is, until you are satisfied with your hours of sleep. Remember to be realistic here. Don't expect eight hours a night if you are 80, inactive and have never been a good sleeper.

This strategy sounds rather punishing and it may make you feel worse for a while, but if your sleep problem is difficult to sort out, it's worth trying for a while. Try to stick with it if you can, at least for a month or two, unless you feel that it's clearly working in the wrong direction. Things may have to feel a little bit worse for a while before they get better, but only a little bit. Sleep restriction is frequently used by sleep clinics to good effect.

It may be worth re-reading this section to make sure you're clear how this strategy works.

If you feel very alone with this, it can be useful to share it with someone, a friend, partner or whoever. Not sleeping is a miserable and lonely experience. If you find that this technique is making you feel much worse, stop using it and, particularly if you are feeling very low in mood or having black or self-destructive thoughts, go to see your GP.

Paradoxical injunction

If sleep restriction is somewhat counter-intuitive, this strategy is completely so; that's the whole point of it. It means trying to do the opposite of what you're after, or seeming to do so.

At its simplest, this means going to bed and not trying to sleep – in fact, trying *not* to sleep but to rest. It makes good sense for many, because trying so hard to sleep is often what keeps you awake. By removing the effort to sleep, arousal falls and sleep will often ensue. Isn't it so often the way with life, that things happen just when you don't need them to, when you're not trying?

A refinement on this technique which I like is to timetable your least favourite chore, not involving strenuous physical or mental effort, for 2 a.m. Every student knows that when it's time to revise, you feel sleepy. You settle down in the afternoon for a good few hours of study and promptly doze off. It's ridiculous – any other time you'd never sleep in the afternoon. But it isn't: your brain is doing what it does. It is switching off from what it doesn't want to do, so in response to the grinding prospect of hours of study, the SCN switches off and you fall asleep.

You can use this phenomenon. My least favourite task is ironing; it's really tedious. So for me, if I needed to use paradoxical injunction, I would timetable the ironing for 2 a.m. If I'm awake then, at least I get a job done and I'm not lying in bed fretting about not sleeping. As likely as not, though, the prospect of this irksome chore will send me to sleep.

There are many variations on this theme. The bottom line is the one I keep coming back to: *stop trying to sleep*.

11

Pills and potions

It's a funny thing. Most people who I see in my consulting room complaining of insomnia are on sleeping pills (hypnotics) of one kind or another. That's natural, I hear you say, but I don't think so. Very few have been advised to try any of the measures which I have outlined in the last three chapters. I think that's a shame, as the available evidence suggests that, in people with enduring sleep problems, psychological and behavioural methods and treatments work at least as well as medications over a whole population. They don't have side effects, they aren't addictive and their effect is lasting, while medications only work for as long as you take them. It seems that adding sleeping tablets to a treatment regime involving the measures which I listed doesn't improve the overall efficacy of the treatment package. In fact, there is a suggestion that sleeping tablets may render treatment less successful on some occasions. This would not be surprising, as relying on a pill to send you to sleep is likely to distract you from your efforts to get good at relaxation, mindfulness, stress management, sleep hygiene and other effective sleep-promoting strategies. I'm not blaming GPs for this, as there really isn't time in a primary care consultation to go through the sorts of measures contained in this book and they are under a lot of pressure to provide solutions to the problems presented to them. It is a shame, though, that basic sleep advice isn't pushed a bit more by the National Health Service. Chemical-free measures to tackle insomnia work for many and I don't think that pills should be your first port of call.

I have experienced pressure to prescribe myself, on many occasions. It seems ironic to me that most people would not consider taking tranquillizers long term, because we all know that to do so risks addiction, but many of us are more than happy to take a sleeping tablet every night – indeed, some of my patients insist on it. I fully understand this, as insomnia is horrible. But a sleeping tablet is a tranquillizer at higher dosage. Take a tranquillizer and increase the dose threefold and you'll fall asleep. All right, I accept that there are some subtle differences between the mode of action of the sleeping tablets most commonly used today (the z-drugs; see page 72) and the tranquillizers (Valium, Librium and Ativan) which were demonized in the 1980s and 90s, but, as I will go on to explain in this chapter, there are similarities too. Beware any pill which holds out the promise of a risk-free long-term solution to anxiety or insomnia. Taking sleeping tablets long term may cause more problems than are solved.

Having said all of this, I occasionally prescribe sleeping tablets and the other sleep-promoting medicines which I will list in this chapter. They can sometimes be very useful for specific purposes in short-term use, after careful consideration of the pros and cons of using them and of the need to do so. I also take one myself on an occasional basis (zopiclone), prescribed by my GP. As I mentioned earlier, I spend most of my holidays in the USA. I take one tablet the first night that I'm there, to get into the new time zone, one on the plane home (it's a red-eye flight) and one on the first night back. That's usually fewer than ten tablets a year, which doesn't pose a significant risk of addiction and it works very well. That is the sort of situation in which sleeping pills can be useful. Taking them for months or years as the sole measure to tackle insomnia, however, is in my opinion usually counter-productive. Some doctors recommend taking sleeping tablets for a few nights 'to re-establish a sleeping pattern'. I don't know of any evidence that this works and in my experience the sleep problem tends to re-emerge as soon as the drug is stopped, but there's no harm in trying it, I suppose, so long as you really do stop the drug after a few days. In practice this can be difficult to do.

If you have been on a sleeping tablet for years, don't suddenly stop it, as you will very likely suffer withdrawal symptoms, prime among them being insomnia, which is the last thing you need right now. Seek the advice of your GP first of all and don't panic. It is possible to get off sleeping tablets, but you need to do so on medical advice and gradually. There are a few people who need to remain on sleeping tablets long term. So long as this is on medical advice, under medical supervision, with no escalation of dosage over time, it need not lead to major problems. The trouble is that, in my experience, many long-term users of sleeping tablets take them without regular medical review and are psychologically dependent on them. With the older sleeping tablets, escalation of dosage is common, though it is much less so with the newer z-drugs.

All right, lecture over. As I've said, sedative drugs can be useful in short-term use for specific situations. Let's have a look at the various different types now.

Benzodiazepines

These drugs, such as nitrazepam and temazepam, used to be the mainstay of insomnia treatment. They fell out of fashion when it was found that some users were getting addicted to them. This involved needing steadily higher doses, craving the drug and experiencing a serious rebound worsening of insomnia when coming off. Temazepam became increasingly popular among drug addicts, with an increasing street value. As they are of the same class of drugs as diazepam (Valium), chlordiazepoxide (Librium) and lorazepam (Ativan), when these tranquillizers fell off their pedestal during the 1980s with scary stories of thousands of people getting addicted, the equivalent sleeping tablets also fell out of favour. However, they are still occasionally used today.

Benzodiazepine hypnotics work on GABA, the sedative trans- mitter chemical in the brain (see Chapter 2), increasing the firing of nerves triggered by it. This system of nerves promotes relaxation, relief of anxiety and, at higher levels, sleep. So benzodiazepine hypnotics are effective at promoting sleep in the short term. Unfortunately, the brain tends to resist any change you try to make to it, so in longer-term use the brain tends to switch itself on again in opposition to the effect of the drug. Then when the hypnotic is stopped, the brain is even more aroused than it was before the drug was started, so sleep is worse than ever, at least for a while. These withdrawal effects are temporary, so if this rebound insomnia is tolerated by a gritting of the teeth for a while, sleep does eventually come back to how it was before the hypnotic was started.

Another problem with benzodiazepine hypnotics is that they alter sleep architecture. They tend to increase time spent in stage 2 of sleep, while reducing time in the more restorative deeper stages 3 and 4 and sometimes abolishing REM sleep altogether. This isn't ideal in terms of promoting well-being.

In addition, benzodiazepines tend to be longer acting than the z-drugs, so there is a greater risk of hangover effects with them, and they should not be used by those with sleep apnoea as they can reduce the respiratory drive, potentially increasing the time during which breathing stops, which could pose a potential risk in this condition (there is no risk of this in people who don't have sleep apnoea).

No surprise, then, that they have been largely superseded by the z-drugs. Nonetheless, benzodiazepine hypnotics are perfectly good drugs for short-term use

The z-drugs

These newer sleeping pills work on the same receptors in the brain as the benzodiazepines, also increasing GABA activity, but they do so rather more subtly and so carry some advantages over the older compounds. In particular, tolerance (reduced effect over time leading to dosage escalation) occurs much more slowly and in many cases apparently not at all. They seem to alter sleep architecture much less than benzodiazepines, allowing some time in the deeper stages 3 and 4 of sleep (though these deeper stages are still reduced compared to non-drug-induced sleep) and often some REM sleep too. While rebound insomnia when the drug is stopped does occur, the severity of this withdrawal effect tends to be less than for the benzodiazepines, and it seems that it is no worse when a regular user comes off after several years compared to someone withdrawing after a few months. These drugs have virtually no street value. This is not to say that there is no risk of getting dependent on z-drugs; there is, but the risk is less. If you are using them long term, the risk can be minimized by not using the drug every night and employing 'drug holidays': that is, spells of several days when you don't take a pill, for example on holiday or when not sleeping well isn't so important.

There is some evidence that improving sleep as quickly as possible can speed up recovery from depressive illness in some people, so the z-drugs may be prescribed for a limited period together with an antidepressant early in treatment of a depressive episode.

Z-drugs also don't have much of an anti-anxiety effect and so don't promote psychological dependence as powerfully as the benzodiazepines. I know this lack of tranquillizing effect from personal experience. When I first took a zopiclone tablet on the night flight back from Atlanta to London, it didn't seem to be working. After about half an hour I turned to my wife and said: 'This drug is useless. It doesn't ...' The sentence was never completed and six hours later I woke up.

The potential problem of dependence is lower the longer acting the drug is. The longest acting of the z-drugs presently available in the UK is zopiclone (Zimovane), the next longest is zolpidem (Stilnoct) and the shortest acting is zaleplon (Sonata).

If your problem is getting to sleep but once asleep you tend not to wake up, a shorter-acting drug is probably right for you as it gets you to sleep quickly but is out of your system within a few hours. If you get to sleep but wake up too early, then a longer-acting one is preferable, as it needs to be still in your system at the time you have been waking up. If you wake at, say, 3 a.m. some nights and can't get back to sleep, there is an argument for taking a short-acting z-drug when you wake up, as sometimes you won't need it, reducing the risk of dependence, and it is less likely to cause a hangover. It is worth pointing out here what is hopefully obvious: if you wake up drowsy and still under the influence of the sleeping tablet, you shouldn't drive. In selecting the appropriate z-drug, again your sleep diary is a useful reference point.

One problem which may be greater for longer-acting z-drugs may particularly affect the elderly. If the drug does not lead to you falling asleep, you are likely nonetheless to be somewhat drugged and disorientated, leading to an increased risk of falls and other accidents if you get up in the night. For this reason, if the medication doesn't work to get you to sleep, it may be wise to stop taking it, but if you do, tell your GP.

Of people who take zopiclone, 40 per cent get an unpleasant metallic taste from it. This is a genetically inherited trait, so if you get it, it will always taste that way.

Sedative antihistamines

These drugs are widely used and are available over the counter, without prescription. They include diphenhydramine (Nytol) and promethazine (Phenergan). They are also present in a lot of cold and flu remedies (such as Night Nurse).

Antihistamines have a low addictive potential and people don't often seem to escalate the dose. However, they are rather long-acting, tending to leave you feeling drugged the next day (beware driving or operating heavy machinery) and the evidence for their efficacy in any but mild and transient insomnia is scanty. If you take one of these remedies regularly, be sure to tell your GP, as they do interact with a number of prescribed medicines.

Sedative antidepressants

The good thing about antidepressants is that they aren't addictive. That is, they seem to maintain their effect well at a constant dose and don't tend to lead to dosage escalation or to craving. They can cause withdrawal effects if stopped abruptly, but as they tend to be taken at low dosage when used exclusively to treat insomnia, this tends not to be a problem in practice. It can be when they are taken at higher dosage to treat insomnia secondary to major depression, but this can usually be managed quite easily by withdrawing them slowly when the time comes. Amitriptyline (see below) also has analgesic properties at low dosage (10–25 mg), which can be useful if pain is keeping you awake.

Sedative antidepressants don't always work well for severe or long-standing insomnia and they all have potential side effects. For example, mirtazapine (Zispin) can cause a ferocious carbo-hydrate craving leading to weight gain in some and, being long acting, tends to cause drowsiness the next day. Tricyclics such as amitriptyline and trazodone can cause dry mouth, blurred vision, dizziness on standing, constipation or difficulty passing water in some people, and they aren't advised in those with heart disease. They are very dangerous in overdosage, so you must not take more than has been prescribed. Agomelatine (Valdoxan), which works in part on the melatonin system (see page 6), can be useful in some depressed people who are sleeping poorly, but some doctors feel that it may not work for severe depression as often as some other antidepressants (everyone is different in their response to these drugs and the research evidence for the efficacy of agomelatine appears to be sound).

Antipsychotic drugs

Most of the drugs used to treat psychotic illnesses such as schizophrenia are sedative and at low dosage can act as sleeping tablets. However, most can cause weight gain in some and tend to leave you feeling slowed down the next day, so in practice their use is limited, but a few people, particularly those with high levels of anxiety, find them very helpful and they have virtually no addictive potential. Examples are quetiapine (Seroquel) and olanzapine (Zyprexa).

Anti-epileptic drugs

All anti-epileptic drugs are, to a greater or lesser extent, sedative. One in particular, pregabalin (Lyrica), seems to have quite a strong anti-anxiety effect and it has a formal licence in the UK as a treatment for anxiety disorders. Pregabalin and the related anti-epileptic drug gabapentin (Neurontin) also have pain-relieving properties. Both, and particularly pregabalin, have been used to help people with sleep problems where the main reasons for insomnia are anxiety or pain, or both. They don't have a licence for treatment of insomnia, which doesn't mean that they can't be used for this purpose, just that the manufacturers can't advertise them as treatments for sleep difficulties. In practice, though, few GPs would be comfortable prescribing drugs of this sort outside their licensed indication and they are really only prescribed for insomnia by psychiatrists and specialist sleep clinics.

Melatonin

You already know about the role of this hormone, naturally produced by the body, in promoting sleep (see Chapter 2). Essentially, it is the substance which switches your lights off, turning off the SCN and thus switching on the sleep response. It can be taken in pill form, as a slow-release preparation under the trade name Circadin, and it has a UK licence for treatment of insomnia, but only in those aged over 55. This is because the strongest evidence for its efficacy is in older people, which isn't surprising as the body's production of melatonin slows with age. Essentially, some older people may be deficient in this hormone, resulting in them not having an effective switch to turn off the SCN. This is one of the reasons that insomnia is commoner in older people.

Melatonin is taken one or two hours before bedtime. It isn't particularly sedative, but it does help in some people to reset a normal circadian rhythm, and means that going to sleep and waking up happen at a time close to when they used to occur. While this isn't what it's licensed for, it is sometimes taken by frequent flyers to get them into the new time zone, reducing jet lag, and also by shift workers, who have to cope with frequently changing sleep–wake times. It isn't supposed to be taken for more than 13 weeks, the idea being that by this time your internal circadian rhythm will have been reset effectively. I'm not sure about this logic, particularly in the elderly, and I know that some people do take it for longer than this, though I can't recommend it.

Melatonin is a relatively recent addition to the UK hypnotic market. There aren't any major worries about it at this stage, though it shouldn't be taken by anyone with significant liver problems and, like all medicines, it has side effects in some. I intuitively have a slight concern about it, though I can't back this up with any evidence at this stage. In general, if one gives a person a hormone in tablet form for an extended period, that person's own internal production of the hormone decreases. The body has feedback mechanisms in place and recognizes when sufficient of the hormone is present, so if you load up with the hormone taken from an external source, the body will tend to switch off production. It could be that taking melatonin in the long run could stop you producing it. I must make clear that this phenomenon has never to date been demonstrated with melatonin, but then problems with medicines sometimes do take a while to emerge. It does appear, as far as we can tell, that melatonin taken for 13 weeks or less is fairly safe, though in my experience it doesn't work for everyone. Anecdotally, some colleagues have patients who have been on melatonin for much longer than this without problems.

Herbal remedies

If you've read any of my other books, you'll know that these and other 'alternative' treatments are my bugbear. They are popular because they are 'natural'. Why a drug should be better because it comes from a plant escapes me. It certainly doesn't make it safer, as these compounds haven't gone through the same level of rigorous evaluation which is demanded of pharmaceutical preparations. Some of the most toxic substances known to man come from plants, though I'm not suggesting that herbal sleeping remedies are toxic.

The herb valerian is included in most alternative and herbal sleeping draughts and tablets. It seems relatively safe, with a low addictive potential, but is usually ineffective in any but the mildest short-term sleep problems. It interacts (like all pharmaceutical hypnotics) with other sedative drugs, including alcohol. It can also alter the metabolism by the liver of some other medicines, so make sure your GP knows if you're taking it. There are a number of other herbs which can be slightly helpful in some, such as camomile, hops and lemon balm.

So in terms of herbal sleep remedies, there isn't any scientific evidence for their efficacy, but that doesn't mean that they can't work for an individual. Doing a therapeutic trial of one – that is, trying it and seeing if it works for you – can be good science. As you can tell, though, I'm not generally very impressed by herbal preparations. If they work for you, fair dos; everyone is different.

This list of hypnotics isn't exhaustive, but it covers most of the main classes of drugs. My description of their effects, side effects and interactions is certainly way short of being comprehensive because there is limited space in this book. Always seek the advice of your doctor about any medications, these included. In general, short-term use of sleeping tablets is fine, but long-term use tends to make the problem worse. The trouble is that it is very difficult to stop taking a pill which initially gives you a good night's sleep. Try to look at this issue in the long term if you can, though I know it's difficult as sleeplessness is so miserable. Please don't use sleeping tablets as the only treatment of your insomnia.

12

Dealing with specific causes of insomnia

So we've dealt with some of the things you can do to sleep better, whatever the cause of your insomnia. There are, however, some specific conditions linked to poor sleep, as I described in Chapters 4 and 6, for which you need to take particular measures. They are in some ways easier to deal with than idiopathic insomnia (where we don't know the cause or where it's down to stress), because successful treatment of the underlying condition often leads to the sleep problem righting itself. Not always though, because once insomnia starts, anxiety about not sleeping tends to maintain it, regardless of how long ago the original cause was resolved. On a more positive note, the converse may also be true: even if the condition is chronic, sleep can be improved by doing the right things.

Physical illnesses

Many of the things which improve chronic physical illnesses also improve sleep. For example, exercise, taken moderately following medical advice, is an important part of recovery from most conditions, including cardiovascular disease, diabetes, respiratory disorders and most pain syndromes. It also helps you sleep, as I've already pointed out.

When you're laid up with a long-term illness, you need to create a pattern and texture to your life in order to sleep well, but also to maintain the morale which a long recovery process requires. This means finding some routines, some things to look forward to and some demands on yourself and your body. The demands may be mental, such as reading a book or doing a crossword, or may be physical, like struggling into the kitchen to make a cup of tea rather than always having it brought to you. What you need to avoid, if at all possible, is just lying in bed for day after day being a patient. If that's unavoidable and what you're told by the doctors you need to do, so be it, but if not, try to introduce some activity into your life, as it will improve both your sleep and your morale.

Many physical illnesses respond well to psychological treatments such as relaxation training, CBT and mindfulness (see Chapter 9). If you get good at these techniques, both your physical illness and your sleep are likely to improve. Irritable bowel syndrome (IBS) particularly comes to mind as a condition which can respond wonderfully well to these types of treatment, leading in turn to much less disturbed nights.

Anything which helps pain is going to improve sleep, so long as it is neither stimulant nor addictive. There are a variety of excellent TENS (Transdermal Electrical Neurone Stimulation) machines on the market which are very helpful for many people suffering from some chronically painful conditions. Check with your GP for advice before getting one. They work by creating a tingling sensation on the skin in the area above the source of the pain. As skin sensation tends to travel to the spinal cord faster than sensation from deeper structures, this tingling tends to shut the 'gate' on the pain from those structures, rather like rubbing your skin over an area of your body which has suffered a painful blow.

Some medications have multiple actions, for example being analgesic, sedative and anxiety-reducing, thus killing a number of birds with one stone. Examples, as I outlined in Chapter 11, are the antidepressant amitriptyline and the anti-epileptic drug pregabalin, both often used by pain clinics to treat chronic pain, while also promoting sleep and tending to reduce anxiety. On the other hand, as I described earlier, some medicines interfere with sleep in some people through being stimulant, causing vivid dreaming or other disruption of sleep architecture, or through causing a reversal of their own sedative effect over time (a problem with all potentially addictive drugs). It's worth checking with your doctor that none of your medicines could be contributing to your insomnia, and if they are, whether there is an alternative which is less likely to impair sleep.

Mental illnesses

This term is really a misnomer when discussing major or clinical depression (depressive illness), which is a physical illness, not a mental illness, involving a real chemical disturbance in the brain and hormonal changes in the body. It's this illness which I'm going to focus on in this section as sleep problems caused by anxiety disorders are largely dealt with in Chapter 8 and treatment of other mental illnesses such as psychotic disorders is beyond the scope of this book.

People with clinical depression tend to wake early in the morning and not be able to get back to sleep, though sometimes they also have difficulty getting to sleep (a symptom of anxiety) because depression and anxiety tend to go together. Most people with anything more than a mild episode of depression would be well advised to go on to an antidepressant medication. While this isn't the long-term answer to depression, it is essential first aid. Your GP will be able to advise on whether you need an antidepressant, and if you want more information on the subject, have a look at my book *Depressive Illness: The curse of the strong* (Sheldon, 2012). If insomnia is a major symptom of your depression it needs to be treated effectively as otherwise a vicious cycle is set up, with depression causing the insomnia which stops the depressive illness healing. The best choice would be to go on to a sedative antidepressant such as mirtazapine (Zispin), amitriptyline (Triptizol) or agomelatine (Valdoxan) (see Chapter 11). The last of these is only mildly sedative, but working in part on the melatonin system is purported to improve the circadian rhythm, effectively resetting your sleep clock. This may be a better way than pure sedation of improving sleep in some people, as the more sedative drugs may leave you drowsy the next morning, which isn't a good idea if you drive to work.

Some experts recommend taking one of the z-drugs for a while to deal with the insomnia caused by major depression, as there is some evidence that effectively restoring sleep hastens recovery from depression and these medications are probably the quickest to achieve this. As you will have gathered, though, it isn't my favourite strategy as some people will become dependent on them, and struggling to get off a sleeping tablet isn't really what you need when you're trying to recover from depression. If you do go on a z-drug, zopiclone is probably the best option, being the least addictive and sufficiently long-acting to get you past the characteristic early morning waking pattern of depressive illness, though a few people take the ultra-short-acting zaleplon not last thing at night but when they wake up, as it is only active for a few hours and so causes no appreciable hangover effect.

Exercise, which as I've already explained helps promote sleep if taken moderately at the right time, is also an antidepressant, so all the more reason to start a gently graded fitness programme.

CBT is a lot more available now under the NHS and is an effective treatment for depression, having a much more enduring effect than antidepressants alone. Essentially, antidepressants get you better and CBT keeps you better. If you are offered CBT for your depression, ask your therapist to spend a session or two on your insomnia, as CBT for insomnia works (see Chapter 9).

In my view the most important factor in recovery from major depression is understanding it. This is the physical illness which happens to the best people, those who try too hard and give too much. Learning how to pull back a bit, to pace yourself, to find a balance, to learn how to rest effectively, to focus on your own needs as well as those of others, to work out what you want from your life: these are the lessons which help you get better and prevent you getting ill again in the future. If you can find the answers, they will also do a lot to help you sleep well.

Jet lag

This is a time-limited condition, lasting on average one day for every time zone crossed, so many people don't treat it at all, just waiting for it to pass. However, frequent travellers, those who have high-pressure jobs in which they have to function well as soon as they arrive in the new country and those who want to avoid the risk of temporary insomnia for one reason or another, all tend to need a solution to the problem of jet lag.

I've already disclosed my solution, a zopiclone tablet for one or two nights in the new time zone. It works well for me, but doesn't seem to work so well for some others. Jet lag isn't just about not sleeping. It is a disturbance of your whole circadian rhythm and can affect pretty much every function of your brain and body. For this reason, many people find that taking melatonin for a few nights after travelling works better, as this tends to reset your body clock, persuading your nervous system that it really is the time the clock says rather than whatever time it is back home. Logically, this should work best for west to east travel, as you shouldn't need melatonin to get you to sleep when you've been awake for 24 hours or so after a long journey east to west, and in tending to shift your circadian rhythm forward melatonin is actually working in the wrong direction. In practice some people take it in both directions of travel. Melatonin should only be taken on medical advice. It is available over the counter in some countries, but I wouldn't advise using it without a doctor advising on its use. In the UK it's usually prescribed in slow-release form (Circadin).

It's also worth attending to the other factors which affect your circadian rhythms. For example, if you are due to travel to the west coast of America, say Los Angeles (eight hours behind the UK), it is worth, if possible, slowly shifting your routine for a week or so prior to travel, taking your meals gradually later, going to bed gradually later and, if it's an option, getting up gradually later. Try to have lights, LCD screens and the like on as brightly as possible later in the evening than normal and keep your curtains tightly closed later than you normally would in the morning. Then when you get to LA, go to bed fairly early in the evening to begin with, gradually moving your bedtime later over a few days, but don't take a nap as soon as you arrive at your destination. Wait until (early) bedtime. Get up with the dawn at first (though keeping the curtains closed) and then gradually move your time of rising to your normal get-up time over the same period. Likewise, try to move mealtimes and other regular habits to the new time zone gradually. If you can't go to bed early in the new time zone, having light fairly bright early in the evening will tend to delay the onset of sleepiness.

When you return to the UK, the exact reverse procedure pertains. Prior to travel move mealtimes and other habits forward, go to bed progressively earlier, get up earlier, put the lights on brightly in the morning but have them dimmed in the evening. Then when you get to the UK go to bed late and (if possible) get up late, again with bright lights in the morning and as little light as possible in the evening, gradually shifting to a normal pattern over a few days.

While this type of strategy won't be possible for everyone (business doesn't wait for your body clock), the nearer you can get to it the less you'll suffer from jet lag.

Whatever else you do, it seems that regular exercise, again not too near bedtime, helps to minimize the effects of jet lag in many. Also remember that the principles of not drinking coffee, tea or a lot of alcohol too near bedtime get shifted to the new time zone. A couple of cups of coffee on the plane just before it lands, though taken at what feels like first thing in the morning, may be near enough to the end of the UK day to interfere with sleep. In any case, it's best not to drink a lot of alcohol or caffeine on the plane. Drink plenty of water, though. On a night flight, use an eye mask and earplugs.

Be understanding with yourself. However hard you try, you probably won't be at your best for a few days after a long journey around the world.

Shift work

The problems here are similar to those involved in jet lag, involving shifts in your circadian rhythm, but unlike those engaging in occasional trips to distant shores, many on shift work have to get used to a new sleep–wake cycle every few days. The principles of how to manage it are similar, though, starting with recognizing that *shift work is hard* and you can't expect yourself to perform as well in a frequently changing shift pattern including night-time shifts as you would if working a consistent 9 to 5. Yes, by all means show this paragraph to your boss if you think it'll make her more understanding … no, I didn't think so.

Because your sleep pattern is impacted every few days, taking a sleeping tablet really isn't often an option, unless you only change to or from a night shift once a month or less. Melatonin for a day or two, taken an hour or so before bedtime (that is in the morning after the night shift), should theoretically tend to pull forward the time you get to sleep. When you come off the night shift, taking melatonin in the evening should tend again to bring forward sleep onset. Equally, taking melatonin as soon as you wake up for a few mornings tends to lead to you sleeping later and then staying awake later, but in practice this effect is rarely used. In any case, the results of research into the efficacy of melatonin in shift-work induced insomnia have been unimpressive.

As with jet lag, attending to your regular habits, shifting them gradually towards your new sleep–wake pattern before the new shift pattern starts, is worthwhile. When you start a night shift, try to ensure that light is as bright as possible from when you get up and particularly early in the shift. A full-spectrum light source may be a good investment. On the drive home, you may find it helpful to wear dark glasses, so long as this doesn't impair your vision or driving ability. Then, when you get home, try to keep things quiet if possible (if you haven't got children!), close the curtains wherever you are for the few hours before bed and make sure that the lights aren't too bright. Keep coffee and tea to the first half of the shift. Avoid heavy meals during the shift if possible. Some people find that a short nap prior to the shift is helpful. While daytime naps usually impair sleep and are not recommended for people with sleep problems, your circadian rhythms are already disrupted by shift work, so this rule can be relaxed if you find a brief pre-shift kip helps.

At weekends, be realistic. Don't try to be there for the kids all through the weekend if you've been doing nights Monday to Friday. Be selective. If your son has a football match on Saturday afternoon, go to that, but sleep right up to midday if you can, then make sure you are in a brightly lit setting for an hour or two before the game.

Bright light early in the morning causes a phase advance of your circadian rhythms (see Chapter 2 and above), bringing forward your period of wakefulness and also bringing forward the time later in the day when you feel sleepy. The same light in the evening causes a phase delay: that is, delaying the onset of sleepiness and making it likely that you'll go to sleep later and sleep until later in the morning. You can use this principle to manipulate your sleep–wake cycle, but only to an extent. There is a limit to the power of light.

Restless leg syndrome (RLS)

This is a miserable affliction, described in Chapter 6, at its worst when you're in bed hoping to sleep. It is common, affecting around 5 per cent of the population, and so is one of the major causes of insomnia. As I explained, many people with depressive illness will need to be on antidepressant medication. Unfortunately most of these drugs can cause or worsen RLS. Mirtazapine and venlafaxine are reputed to be particular culprits. If you are on an antidepressant and are afflicted with this condition, a reduction in dosage or a change of antidepressant may be required. Some people have to change drug regularly to avoid the symptoms emerging. If you have RLS, don't take an antihistamine to help you sleep as it is likely to make the symptoms worse.

There are other causes of restless legs and sometimes there's no cause; it tends to run in families. It is worth checking that you don't have iron deficiency, though, as that can be a cause; it is easily checked by a blood test and equally easily treated by taking an iron supplement.

Reducing alcohol and caffeine consumption can help a great deal, as can taking a hot bath and/or doing a calf muscle-stretching exercise before bedtime. Check with your doctor if you have any physical problems which might make stretching difficult or hazardous. I tend to restless legs myself and I find that hanging my heels off a step, holding on to a banister or the wall, for about 30 seconds to a minute is very helpful. A physiotherapist will give more detailed advice if you need it.

In general, regular exercise reduces the severity of restless leg syndrome, but again, not too near bedtime.

If nothing else works, there are medications called dopamine agonists, such as rotigotine (Neupro), which are helpful for some people. They sometimes lose their effect over time, with the symptoms coming back worse than ever. This effect is minimized by using as low a dose as possible and switching to another drug at the first sign of it occurring. If these drugs don't work, don't despair: there are a number of other medications which can help, including some of the anti-epileptic drugs such as pregabalin and gabapentin.

As RLS tends to go together with involuntary movements during sleep, this is one of those conditions in which it may be worth sleeping in a separate bed from your partner or spouse for a while, until you've had some success in dealing with it. This avoids the unhappy cycle of taking ages to get to sleep, only to have him angrily wake you up a short while later because your restlessness is keeping him awake, then leaving you awake with your restless legs while he happily snores the night away. Sometimes being practical about sleeping arrangements can protect the romance in your relationship better than always sleeping together.

Sleep apnoea

The most important measure to take if you are overweight and have sleep apnoea is to lose weight. You need to get into the weight range which gives you a body mass index (BMI) of 20–25. BMI is defined as weight in kilograms divided by height in metres squared (i.e. height multiplied by itself). So if you weighed 100 kg and were 2 metres tall (about 6 ft 8 in), your BMI would be $100/2 \times 2 = 100/4 = 25$. Achieving this through a healthy diet and exercise may well fix the problem.

Making sure that any upper respiratory disease such as bronchitis or asthma is treated effectively may also be important. If you smoke, do your best to give up. If the problem emerges after the menopause, HRT may be indicated. Discuss this with your GP.

Alcohol tends to cause relaxation of the muscles of the pharynx and so is best avoided. If you do drink, do so only very moderately, keeping it to one small drink once or twice a week. Most sleeping tablets, in particular the benzodiazepines such as nitrazepam and temazepam (in fact anything ending in 'pam') are muscle relaxants and should also be avoided if possible.

Again, as with RLS, there may be an argument for sleeping separately from your partner, probably in a different room if one is available. I know I'm sounding like an unromantic spoilsport, but there's nothing romantic about chronic sleep deprivation for both of you. If you are sleeping with someone with sleep apnoea, he or she isn't going to suffocate in the night. It's not to say that the condition does no harm; it's definitely not good for you in the long term, but you don't need to worry that it will lead to death from asphyxia tonight. Assuming your partner doesn't have any other medical condition, the drive to breathe is very strong and will prevail in the end.

If these measures don't work, you may need to be fitted for a jaw splint. This pulls your jaw forward while you sleep, thus helping to keep the airways open. Another possible solution is a CPAP (Continuous Positive Airway Pressure) device. This is a mask which covers your face with an airtight seal, linked to a supply of air delivered at a moderately high pressure. This positive air pressure can help to prevent the airway from collapsing in the deep stages of sleep, as it tends to in sleep apnoea. These devices are a bit cumbersome and don't work for everyone, but for some they are very effective.

There are surgical interventions which have been used for sleep apnoea. They are worth avoiding except as a last resort. I'm not an expert in these operations, but I think most people are agreed they have disadvantages and certainly should not be your first port of call.

If simple measures such as weight loss and stopping drinking alcohol don't solve the problem, your next step is to talk to your GP before deciding what to do next.

13

I still can't sleep

So you've done everything suggested in this book so far, but still your sleep is poor. What next?

The answer is to keep going. Many of the strategies which I have listed take a lot of practice to become effective. Anything which isn't working tends to make you tense, so I wouldn't expect your sleep to improve straight away. Stick at it and eventually, when the techniques become second nature, they will start to work.

Check your sleep diary, or restart it for a week or two if you've stopped recording it. Are you sure your sleep isn't improving? This is a process and you shouldn't expect consistent or dramatic effects early in the piece. Any shift in your sleep pattern, consistent or not, is progress. Don't demand that you achieve a particular target of hours slept by a particular date. Sleep doesn't respond to edicts from management; it slips back in quietly when you aren't looking. Don't try to nail it down. I see sleep as like birds. You can build a bird table, put out the grain and keep the cats away, but you can't make the birds come to your garden. You can only provide the most favourable possible environment for them; then it's a question of waiting until they arrive. Waiting is something that many of us aren't very good at, but calm, patient waiting is what is needed here.

How good are you at the core skills which will underpin better sleeping, such as relaxation and mindfulness? Do you routinely CBT yourself on a daily basis? It took me over two years of practising for half an hour every single day, come rain or shine, to get as good as I am now at relaxation, but it was worth it. Now it takes me ten seconds to switch on a relaxed state when I need to, so I don't often have difficulty sleeping. You'll probably be quicker at it than me, and in any case it takes much less time than that to get to the point at which you can use the full relaxation exercise effectively at bedtime – only a month or two for the average person. Stick at it. I CBT myself every day (by which I mean challenging unhelpful thoughts which come into my mind), several times on most working days, as there's plenty of opportunity to get anxious in my job. I never let myself get away with ruminating anxiously about anything. I ask myself: 'Why am I anxious, what am I thinking? Is that thought realistic or probable? No. Is there a more realistic thought or more probable outcome? Yes. Do I accept that alternative thought? Yes. Does that make me feel better? Yes.' That process takes 10 to 20 seconds, because it's second nature now as I've done it thousands of times. CBT is a way of life, not just a strategy. Are you living it? If you aren't, practise some more before assuming that your sleep problem is insoluble.

Have you made real changes in your life, effectively allowing yourself to run at a lower level of arousal? If not, what's stopping you? Are there 'givens' in your life which are keeping you over-aroused and stopping you from sleeping well? If so, you may want to re-examine them. What do you want more, the givens which you have imposed on yourself, such as wealth, success and being labelled the perfect parent, or to be healthy, enjoy things more and sleep better? The choice is yours. You can't have it all. Disappointing, that, isn't it? But it's true; accept this and things will get better, including your sleep.

Look again at your sleep pattern. Are you really suffering from insomnia or are you noticing more nowadays that you've never slept for as many hours as other people? Have your hours of sleep gradually reduced over the years? That's normal; it's not insomnia, it's ageing.

If you really have made changes in your life and got as good as you can at the strategies and skills I've outlined in this book but are still suffering from real insomnia – that is, a pattern of reduced sleep leading to daytime drowsiness and impaired functioning – we need to look again at the problem. Something is getting in the way of a normal sleeping pattern and we need to find out what it is. All right, I know that's obvious – there's no need to shout. The point is that the majority of people who don't sleep well are making mistakes which can be easily rectified, but a few have something else going on.

The next step is to check with your GP that you don't have a physical or mental disorder without realizing it. A few questions (I've outlined some of them in Chapter 4) will reveal if you have major depression, which is the biggest single reason for persistent insomnia. A few more questions, a physical examination and possibly a blood test will uncover most of the physical illnesses which may be underlying. It's well worth taking the step of seeing your GP as most of these conditions are easily treated and will lead to greatly improved sleep.

I find that for many people with apparently unexplainable sleep problems, the answer is revealed by an in-depth exploration of their psychodynamics – that is, discovering those past experiences which are resonating with their current experiences (see Chapter 3). If it is so for you, it may be necessary for you to be referred to a psychiatrist to look for one of these hidden causes and eventually to have a course of exploratory psychotherapy (in the past called psychoanalysis). Unfortunately, this form of therapy isn't very easily accessed through the NHS.

I haven't said much about alternative (sometimes called complementary) therapies, other than herbal remedies, in this book. The reason is that there isn't a lot of evidence for their efficacy. This doesn't mean that they won't help you to sleep; they may do so, because everybody is different. It just means that when their effects are measured in scientific research, the results across a whole population of people with sleep problems are unimpressive. This may be because there is only a small effect in most people, or because the results are good but only in a few. Being a scientist, I'm bound by methods which have a solid evidence base, either from research or from wide clinical experience. Asking me about an alternative treatment is like asking a painter and decorator about a Leonardo da Vinci painting. He'll be able to tell you about the paint, but not the art. Complementary medicine is an art, not a science.

Anecdotally, I've known people who have found hypnosis very helpful for insomnia. This wouldn't be surprising, as hypnosis is a state of deep relaxation, which if successfully induced should help get you to sleep. If hypnotic suggestion can help rid you of some of your unhelpful thoughts and beliefs about sleep (see CBT for insomnia, page 53), this should also help. Other treatments which seem to help some are acupuncture, reflexology and massage. Aromatherapy massage in particular has its proponents. Whether a lavender-scented candle or lavender oil on your pillow, which is reputed to have a calming effect, will have the same effect isn't clear. The problem with these methods, I suspect, is that they may induce short-term relaxation, but they are unlikely to deal with the long-term over-arousal which probably underpins your insomnia. Worth a go, though. I know that some people swear by homeopathy, but I'm deeply sceptical about its whole logical basis so I won't comment on it further. Again, though, whatever works for you gets my vote.

If things still aren't any clearer after you have gone through all of these steps, it may be that you need to be referred to a specialist sleep clinic. In these centres you first of all have a history of your sleep problem taken. Take your sleep diary with you, as it may save time. They may first get you to try out any tips which you haven't already tried from the list in this book. If necessary, they will then book you in for a sleep study. This will involve you going along to a sleep laboratory overnight for the staff to investigate your sleep pattern at first hand.

The sleep lab staff will hook you up to an EEG overnight. This bit of kit involves electrically sensitive pads being attached to various places on your scalp. No needles are involved and the process is painless. The EEG will accurately track your progression through the various stages of sleep, revealing not only your total sleep hours (which as I've mentioned may be more than you think), but also if you are spending too much or too little time in any of the sleep stages.

The team will probably take a video recording of you, covering the whole night. Other parameters, such as your breathing, pulse and blood pressure, may also be monitored. Through these measurements and observations they will be able to build up a detailed picture of your sleep pattern, to define the nature of your sleep disturbance, to rule out phenomena such as sleep apnoea and, based on this data, to develop a modified plan with you for how to improve your sleep.

If you have already taken the measures suggested in this book, it will save a lot of time in the sleep clinic getting to the heart of the problem and finding the right solutions for you.

14

So that's it?

So that's it, then? Is that all I've got? No magic bullets, no panaceas, no new wonder drug, no guarantees of a quick and easy perfect method of sleeping well without the need to put any time in or to make any inconvenient changes in your life? Well, no, sorry. And don't believe anyone who tells you otherwise. There are a lot of snake oil salesmen in this field all too ready to provide you with a quick fix, for a price. Give them a wide berth.

But the good news is that the great majority of people who sleep poorly can sleep better if they persevere with the measures which I've outlined. Stick to the mainstream methods with persistence and you'll have the best chance of getting there in the end.

So let's return to our generic insomniac, Jane, from the introduction. What could she do differently to improve her sleep?

1 *Keep things in proportion* Jane has magnified the consequences of a poor night's sleep so much that it has terrified her. She has thus created a state of over-arousal incompatible with sleep. The truth is that she will get by tomorrow even without much sleep, if she can challenge her thinking sufficiently to be able to spend the night resting. No catastrophe will occur. If necessary, she could share her fears with a sensible friend who can help her to gain a more accurate perspective on things. If she keeps thinking in this type of unhelpfully catastrophic way day after day, she may need to see a cognitive therapist or read a self-help CBT book.

2 *Work on being mindful* If Jane can accept her anxiety and her wakefulness, experiencing them rather than wrestling with them, staying present rather than dealing in self-recrimination for what she feels she's done wrong, leaving tomorrow to tomorrow rather than predicting how awful it will be, then at worst she'll have a restful night of wakefulness and be a whole

lot better off than if she spends the night worrying. At best, the more relaxed state which this mindful approach creates may lead to her sleeping. If she accepts that she can't make herself sleep, sleep will as likely as not arrive in its own time. If she needs to, she could read a book on mindfulness.

3 *Keep to her usual routine* Jane should take her usual early evening jog, as it's early enough not to interfere with sleep, but she should skip the last-minute prep of her presentation, as this raises her arousal level. Most importantly, she should go to bed at the normal time, read her novel as she usually does for ten minutes at bedtime, then turn the light off. These measures will help her to keep in her usual circadian rhythm.

4 *Avoid stimulants (caffeine in her case) after midday* Though there may still be a bit of caffeine in her system at bedtime because of its long duration of action, there won't be enough to interfere with sleep.

5 *Take a bath and a hot milky drink before bedtime* So long as this isn't the only time she takes these measures, they help to promote sleep. Jane shouldn't do anything unusual on, or unique to, this particular night as that will only raise her arousal level.

6 *Stop looking at the clock* Sleep will come when it's ready, not when the clock says it should, so clock-watching is pointless. Jane should turn the clock away from her.

7 *Get up after half an hour or so* As I said earlier, this may seem to contradict point 6, but Jane needs to use a bit of common sense. If she's been awake for what she thinks is over 30 minutes (don't check every few minutes), she can turn the clock round to see if she's right, and if she is she should go to another quiet room and sit in dimmed light, not looking at a screen or doing work (she can take her novel if she wishes) until she feels sleepy. Then she can return to bed, repeating the process in another half an hour or so if she's not asleep.

8 *Write in her repository of thoughts* When the worrying thoughts pop into her head uninvited, Jane should write them roughly (the light is off, so it'll be untidy writing) on the notepad on her bedside table. Then, at the predetermined time in the morning, it's crucial that she looks over these thoughts, however silly

they seem in the cool light of day. It's no excuse for her to say she's too busy to look at her notepad the next morning. Even if she only glances through her list of nocturnal thoughts and dismisses them quickly, she needs to go through this process to enable this strategy to work tomorrow and the next night.

9 *Get good at a relaxation exercise* Jane needs to start practising a relaxation exercise now so that she's good enough at it for it to be useful the next time she's in this situation. She can then use it to help her to sleep and also before her presentation, to avoid having a panic attack like the one which spoiled her last effort. If she has a panic attack anyway, she should accept it and experience it, realizing that a panic attack doesn't harm her and that she can actually carry on with her presentation while it's going on.

10 *Forgive herself for getting it wrong* This is, I think, the most important point of all. If Jane beats herself up for her mistakes she'll never learn from them. She'll just be worried that she's going to mess up again on the next occasion something important comes up, which will make it less likely still that she'll be able to sleep. She did her best, which was all she could have done, given that she didn't have hindsight in advance. Now she knows better and she'll do it differently next time.

Should Jane go to her GP to get a sleeping tablet, in case the need should arise in the future? I don't think so. Jane is someone who pushes herself hard and who tends to get anxious before demanding events. She'll probably do well, and the higher up she gets in her organization, the more of these testing occasions are going to face her. If she relies on taking sleeping tablets before each meeting at which she presents, she's going to get addicted to them. If she does get a prescription for hypnotics, she's going to have to be strict with herself about not taking them regularly. I think it would be a better idea for her to get really good at the other available strategies before going that route, though I accept that a very occasional sleeping tablet is unlikely to do any harm.

So there it is. Sleep is like life, at its best if we take it as it comes and accept its imperfections. Nothing is guaranteed in life and, having practised what I've suggested in this book, you're not guaranteed to sleep well, but I'll tell you what: you're giving yourself the best possible chance of doing so. You'll also probably be happier, because you'll find a better balance in your life. If you continue to struggle with insomnia, your task isn't to defeat it, it's to make the most of the situation you find yourself in. My grandfather was incredibly unlucky at cards, being famed for getting dreadful hands when playing bridge. Rather than bemoaning his ill-fortune, he became the best player of a bad hand who ever lived, or so the story goes. If God gives you lemons, make lemonade.

Working at the strategies in this book may not produce great sleep as promptly as you'd like, but in time it probably will. I'm confident in particular that, if as with most poor sleepers the main cause of your insomnia is stress, doing what I've suggested will get you sleeping much better. But *only when you stop trying to sleep.*

Index